Filling a Need While Making Some Noise

of related interest

Music Therapy in Children's Hospices
Jessie's Fund in Action
Edited by Mercedes Pavlicevic
Foreword by Victoria Wood
ISBN 1 84310 254 4

Music Therapy: Intimate Notes
Mercedes Pavlicevic
ISBN 1 85302 692 1

Clinical Applications of Music Therapy in Developmental Disability,
Paediatrics and Neurology
Edited by Tony Wigram and Jos De Backer
Foreword by Colwyn Trevarthen
ISBN 1 85302 734 0

Music Therapy in Palliative Care
New Voices
Edited by David Aldridge
ISBN 1 85302 739 1

Pied Piper
Musical Activities to Develop Basic Skills
John Bean and Amelia Oldfield
ISBN 1 85302 994 7

Roots of Musicality
Music Therapy and Personal Development
Daniel Perret
Foreword by Colwyn Trevarthen
ISBN 1 84310 336 2

Medical Art Therapy with Children
Edited by Cathy Malchiodi
Foreword by Richard Lippin
ISBN 1 85302 677 8 paperback
ISBN 1 85302 676 X hardback

Filling a Need While Making Some Noise

A Music Therapist's Guide to Pediatrics

Kathy Irvine Lorenzato

Foreword by Kay Roskam

Jessica Kingsley Publishers
London and Philadelphia

First published in 2005
by Jessica Kingsley Publishers
116 Pentonville Road
London N1 9JB, UK
and
400 Market Street, Suite 400
Philadelphia, PA 19106, USA

www.jkp.com

Library of Congress Cataloging in Publication Data
Lorenzato, Kathy, 1955-
    Filling a need while making some noise : a music therapist's guide to pediatrics / Kathy Lorenzato.-- 1st American pbk. ed.
        p. cm.
    Includes bibliographical references (p.   ) and index.
    ISBN-13: 978-1-84310-819-1 (pbk. : alk. paper)
    ISBN-10: 1-84310-819-4 (pbk. : alk. paper) 1. Music therapy for children. I. Title.
ML3920.L84 2005
615.8'5154'083--dc22

                        2005011553

British Library Cataloguing in Publication Data
A CIP catalogue record for this book is available from the British Library

ISBN-10: 1 84310 819 4
ISBN-13: 978 1 84310 819 1

Printed and bound in Great Britain by
Athenaeum Press, Gateshead, Tyne and Wear

*Dedicated to my husband, Stefan, and my children,
MacKenzie and Keenan, without whose love and support
I could not function as a recognizable human being,
much less perform this job.*

To my mother, who believed in me.

"I can't imagine anything but music that could have brought about this alchemy. Maybe it's because music is about as physical as it gets: your essential rhythm is your heartbeat; your essential sound, the breath. We're walking temples of noise, and when you add tender hearts to this mix, it somehow lets us meet in places we couldn't get to any other way."

Anne Lamott, Traveling Mercies

"The art of medicine consists of amusing the patient while nature cures the disease."

Voltaire

Self-portrait

I am made of
memories
held together with
guitar strings
piano wire and
a dozen songs
in the key of D.

Kathy Lorenzato, 2002

Contents

Foreword

Filling a Need While Making Some Noise is a personal and professional diary of the work that Kathy Lorenzato accomplishes as a music therapist in a pediatric unit of a large hospital. In my reading of this book, I felt both touched by the contents, and privileged and grateful to have known Kathy for 20 years as a student, colleague and friend. This book teaches, provides painful insight, and creates awareness and empathy for the patients, families, and caregivers who are living and working every day within a framework of tragedy. This book is also great entertainment. You will laugh and cry, sometimes simultaneously, throughout your reading.

Filling a Need... should be read by anyone who has ever asked the question, "What is music therapy?" It is a must read for all music therapists whether board certified or just entering the field. It should be discussed and thoroughly absorbed by every music therapy student in the 72 training programs in the US. It would also be of great value as a handout to every parent who enters a hospital with his or her ailing child, fearful that "they" – the staff – won't care enough about this child and what he or she may be facing. And it should be read by every health care worker for children (and adults) who questions the incredible worth of their challenging, discouraging, but hopefully gratifying profession.

Filling a Need While Making Some Noise should be continually available to all of the above, and anyone else who happens to come across this book. It is a beautiful reminder of the joys and sorrows that can be expressed through music, of the importance of the best care possible for our children, and for the need to live each day with gratitude for life itself.

Kay Roskam, Ph.D.
Board Certified Music Therapist

Prelude

In my 16-year career at the University of California, Davis Medical Center, I have trained two music therapy interns. While the experience was wonderful and very educational for me, I soon realized that I couldn't keep it up. I am the only music therapist in the hospital, and I work halftime. Plus I have the added benefit of two children at home who are somehow able to sniff out whenever my sick leave exceeds 13 hours and then contract chicken pox, influenza, or scarlet fever, forcing me to stay at home to attend to them and leaving my poor intern alone on Pediatrics. If I have to abandon a seasoned intern, I have no worries. But leaving a new intern on the Pediatric floor can be overwhelming for the intern and gives me guilt. I don't like guilt. I also don't like being pulled in too many different directions.

Before I had interns, I'd entertained the fantasy that the intern would do all the work and I would kick back in the recliner watching soaps on the big screen TV and eating bon-bons. Somehow that fantasy never materialized. As wonderful as both of my interns were (I screened them carefully during the interview process to see if they laughed at my jokes), training them took time away from my patients. It also gave me another layer of responsibility. Not only did I need to make sure my patients were all right, I had to make sure my intern was all right. Working in Pediatrics can be a very intense experience – we're dealing with critically ill children, who are all very beautiful and lovable. It can overwhelm me at times. Interns require a lot of care at the beginning. It became too much for me to balance, so I discontinued the internship.

However, I still get calls and letters asking for internship information. While some are from people who are just desperate and looking every-where for an internship, I know there are a few music therapy students out there who are genuinely interested in working in Pediatrics. There are probably some established music therapists who are interested in venturing into this field as well. I don't blame them. Working on Pediatrics is some of the most fun I've had in my whole life. Other peak experiences include motherhood and riding a bicycle down Haleakala Volcano on the island of Maui, so that's the level of fun I'm talking about here. Just yesterday two nurses told me, "You have the best job in the whole hospital." No contest. I have the most fun in the whole hospital by far! A music therapist would have to be crazy not to love this.

So, since I understand the fun factor of music therapy on Pediatrics, but I cannot provide internships anymore, here is my compromise – a guide for music therapists who want to experience the thrill of working in Pediatrics. This is it – the sum total of all that I feel is important to know. There is no research in this book. There are plenty of research books written about music therapy. As important as research is, experience is equally important. This book is based on what I have learned in my years of working/learning on Pediatrics.

As I told my interns, while I'm sharing some of my tremendous knowledge base with you, your job is to stay awake and nod appropriately. Then before you dutifully do things my way, apply that proverbial grain of salt to everything I've said. I may or may not do everything the way your professors have recommended. What I present here is an approach that has been forged from my own style and background, and it seems to be working for me. You will have your own style and will be in your own institution, abiding by their rules and regulations, and finding your own niche. But trust me on this: Pediatrics is a wonderful place for a music therapist. It is worth volunteering for, fighting for, inservicing[1] on every floor of the hospital for – it is even worth typing six years in the basement for. (See – I knew that degree in piano performance would come in handy someday! I had the fastest fingers around.) However you get into a job in Pediatrics, I promise you will love it.

---

1   Inservice: a short, educational presentation given to a small group. Nearly all the departments in a hospital are required to have several inservices throughout the year, so being the new kid on the block, you'll become very popular and adept at giving these.

A note
on the text

To protect the confidentiality of my patients and their families, all of their names have been changed.

Also, keep in mind that I have MT-BC behind my name, not MD or RN. Medical trends and philosophies seem to change every 20 minutes, so by the time you read this, any medical or nursing observations, or treatment techniques mentioned here may already be obsolete. Hopefully the music therapy observations will endure the test of time on Pediatrics.

1. The Gospel According to Me

I am a music therapist on a pediatric floor, and therefore I am one of the luckiest people in the world. I am paid to make noise and be silly with children. I love my job. It is some of the most fun I've ever had in my life.

For the past 16 years, I have worked in a teaching hospital where the pervasive attitude is one of learning. There are no dumb questions, and education takes place everywhere – in classrooms, hallways, the nurses' stations, and the playroom. There are lots of medical students and nursing students. We have interns in medicine, physical therapy, occupational therapy, speech therapy, respiratory therapy, psychology, Child Life, and sometimes art and music therapy. We even have interns who are chaplains. We teach and learn from all of these people. However, the patients and their families teach all of us the most important lessons – the art of working with children.

Working in pediatrics is wonderful because of the variety of ages (infant through young adult) and complete spectrum of developmental levels it represents. It is also a haven for culture vultures like me. Children come to California from all over the world, representing many languages, cultures and religions. I work with families who have faced extraordinary circumstances: war, refugee camps, giving birth in a jungle, being mauled by a tiger. I am filled with respect for these families who have already been through so much, and now, with a child hospitalized, have yet a new road of hardship to follow. My job is to make that road easier.

1 Goal: fun

Once a patient of ours was admitted to the adult oncology floor because we had no available beds on pediatrics. We'd originally treated him for osteosarcoma (a bone cancer) when he was 17 years old. Now he had recurrence of his tumor at age 21. He certainly qualified as an adult, but since our entire staff was deeply bonded to this young man and his wonderful mom, our pediatric oncology service still followed him. Our oncology resource nurse went up to the adult floor to meet with his mom and told her, "We're trying to get your son back down to the pediatric floor because you both know the nurses and it will be more comfortable for you there."

The mother said, "Thanks. I know he's 21, but we'd prefer to be on pediatrics. Being on this floor is all right, but it's like the difference between church and Disneyland. Up here it's quiet and peaceful – like church. But being on pediatrics is like Disneyland. We'd rather be in Disneyland."

When I heard about this conversation I felt honored to be a member of the pediatric staff. The fact that a 21-year-old man would prefer to be on our floor because we are simply more fun than the adult floor was a tremendous compliment. I guess pediatrics is the "happiest place in the hospital." I also thought, I'm part of that. I help make this place Disneyland.

Long ago, toward the end of my internship, I was working with a group of high functioning inpatients on the psychiatric unit of a local hospital. My supervisor had enough confidence in me by this point to leave me alone with the group periodically. I was comfortable within the setting and familiar with the group members, and somehow our session became outrageously silly. All of us, nurses and patients included, were laughing like – you guessed it – crazy! Although it seemed like we all had a good time, I kept feeling as if I were in trouble. I mean, what if a hospital administrator walked by at that moment? Would he have thought I was 'gasp' *unprofessional?*

Two days later I led the group again, this time with my supervisor, Jim, present. The members clearly wanted to go in the direction of the last group session, and I contorted my face to slyly indicate to them by facial tic and winking that the earlier group had been just a little thing between us, but now that Jim was back we had to be serious again. Jim was also watching my facial contortions and I know he was wondering, "Maybe there's an extra bed on this psych unit for my intern." After the group I confessed my "sin" of silliness to my supervisor, and he made it clear that my feeling of being in trouble was my own problem.

I asked, "But what if an administrator walked by and saw us laughing?"

His response was, "Hmmm, they're laughing. And what is it that most of them are hospitalized for?"

"Clinical depression."

"So do you think that it might be OK for clinically depressed people to laugh?"

"Yeah, I guess that's OK."

He gave me permission to be funny. I have since realized that humor expands the parameters of my practice in a very positive way. And I tell my interns that *fun* is *always* one of our goals on pediatrics.

Now fun has gotten a bad reputation. It's not considered "professional". Somehow the prevailing wisdom says that if you're laughing, you're not working. Well, I'm working at laughing. I take humor very seriously. Norman Cousins wrote two books on the importance of laughing during illness, *Anatomy of an Illness*, and *The Healing Heart*. He believed that he cured himself of ankylosing spondylitis, a progressive and painful inflammatory disease, and recovered from a heart attack by laughing at old-time movies. I'm with him. Laughing always makes me feel better and it seems to help my patients. As humans, we seem to have a biological need to laugh.

Once I was in a room with two 12-year-old girls. A 13-year-old boy came in to join us, and we started telling jokes. Suddenly, all three of these kids yelled, "Wait a minute! Let me get my joke book!" I thought, "You've got to be kidding. You kids thought to bring a joke book to the hospital?" Well, they sure did, and we all fired off jokes for the next 30 minutes. It was wonderful.

On another occasion I was saying goodbye to a 17-year-old woman whom I'd known for a year. She'd undergone treatment for a spinal tumor during all of that time, and although it hadn't progressed, it also hadn't shrunk at all. She was tired of treatment and hospitals and had decided to pursue alternative approaches to her cancer. While we were visiting, we started sharing jokes. Then her oncologist came in, and soon the three of us were taking turns giving our best jokes and laughing together. Now, this doctor is not usually a rollicking bundle of mirth. In fact, he reminds me a lot of Eeyore. But I was so pleased that he was able to join us in a final episode of joint happiness as we said goodbye to a wonderful teenager. We both knew she would probably die in the not too distant future.

Although *fun* is always a goal, people are blessed with silliness to a greater or lesser degree, and if you are not naturally a funny person, do not try this approach! Sometimes people who think they're pretty funny can try too hard with disastrous results. Always focus on the child – let him or her guide you. And do not hesitate to apologize if someone takes your approach the wrong way. Humor also needs to be appropriate. I almost passed out when a doctor told a dirty joke to an eight-year-old in front of his mother and me. Don't tell dirty jokes on pediatrics, even though the teenagers will tell them to you.

You also need to work within the confines of your institution to see what works and what doesn't. Go slowly. I find that I am constantly reinforced for my humor. Once the nurses told me that a gastro-intestinal doctor had read my chart note on a child. I'd written something rather innocuous: "Robbie rocked out in MT [music therapy] group this morning." The doctor laughed out loud when he read it and called all of his residents and medical students over to read it aloud to them. I was amazed at this response, but I keep getting similar reinforcement. Once I attended a multidisciplinary team meeting, and a pulmonologist (lung specialist) said, in front of God and everybody, "The music therapist's chart notes are always appreciated." She didn't say that for anybody else, and I realized I was conditioning these people. They're reading my notes on the chance they may be amused. But the most amazing thing is – they're reading my notes!

It ranks just below the miracle at Lourdes to hear that doctors are taking the time to read the music therapist's notes. These people are fantastically busy. They're also keyed into reading only lab values and tend to skip the "soft, psychosocial issues." But I've been training them slowly by reinforcing them with a laugh if they put in the time to read my notes. It appears that doctors just want to have fun, too.

Lest anyone think that laughter is just entertainment and not real therapy, let me refer them to the piles of research linking humor to the following positive outcomes:

- increased efficiency in the respiratory system (Fry 1977)
- reduced physiological stress response leading to improved clinical outcomes in asthma, heart disease and inflammatory disorders (Hassed 2001)
- enhanced function of the immune system (Dillon and Baker 1986)
- heightened pain threshold (Cogan *et al.* 1987)
- increased positive coping behaviors, even when dealing with anxiety over death (Thorson and Powell 1993)
- elevation of natural killer cell activity – these are lymphocytes (part of the body's immune system) that seek out and kill certain types of cells, including cancer cells (Takahashi *et al.* 2001).

Norman Cousins raised such an interest in the idea that laughter could be beneficial in the treatment of disease that some hospitals have implemented humor programs to be accessible to their patients. Mr Cousins himself was hired at the UCLA School of Medicine in his later years to instruct their students in the therapeutic uses of humor. (I know this because I wrote him a letter in 1987, and he called me on the phone! He was a sweet and personable man – funny, too.) For more on humor programs in hospitals, see the "Resources" section in the back of this book.

Laughter can be contraindicated for patients immediately coming back from surgery. My favorite patients will hold their recent stitches or staples and beg, "Please don't make me laugh!" Of course, the day after surgery, nurses are pushing their patients to breathe into that incentive spirometer[2] in an effort to keep the lungs clear. My feeling is – which would you rather do? Laugh or blow into that little plastic thing? I guarantee one is more fun than the other.

---

2   The incentive spirometer is a plastic device designed to keep patients breathing deeply. They inhale or exhale into the device as hard as they can several times a day. This discourages fluid build-up in the lungs.

2. Is All this Noise Really Necessary? (You Betcha)

In the beginning

A child coming into the hospital has specific needs. Almost universally he or she is afraid. Upon admission nearly every child gets an intravenous (IV) line started, which requires at least one painful poke. Unfortunately, children's veins are notoriously hard to find and tend to roll away from the needle, so any IV start or blood draw may require multiple sticks from even an experienced nurse. Younger children are rarely capable of holding their arm still for such a procedure, so frequently another nurse will help the child remain still by holding them down. From a child's point of view, this looks and feels a lot like torture.

Children (and adults) quickly begin to associate painful procedures with the people who wear white coats or scrubs, so support staff like Child Life specialists and music therapists would not want to dress in the same manner. If you wear white pants, parents will assume you're the nurse and ask, "When is my child being discharged?" Even a white sweater can elicit a fear response in a child. I own an entire collection of oatmeal-colored sweaters – maybe not the most attractive, but at least they don't scare anyone.

Child Life

The specialty of Child Life was developed in response to the problems associated with children in hospitals. Kids can be overwhelmed by the process of hospitalization – the pain, fear, and separation from parents, siblings, and friends, having to stay in a strange and alien environment. They fear exposure and lack of privacy, mutilation, pain, and death. Hospitalization can result in regressive behaviors – bedwetting, thumb sucking, and constant whining – as well as delayed speech, withdrawal, and discipline problems. Some children actually quit talking. Parents once told me their four-year-old son just refused to talk whenever he was in the hospital for his routine chemotherapy. As soon as they pulled up to the driveway of their house, however, he started to jabber again.

We wage a constant battle against depression in any child who's hospitalized for a long period of time. Aggression and violent behaviors may also occur. Forced immobility is not emotionally healthy for anyone, but can really build up rage in a child. I lost my favorite wooden slit drum to a four-year-old boy in traction. He played with such force he actually broke the drum.

The goals of Child Life are to:

1. decrease the trauma and anxiety associated with hospitalization

2. promote normal growth and development, and

3. strengthen coping skills of children and parents (Thompson and Stanford 1950).

Child Life specialists are also experts in child development and do a lot of pre-operative teaching. They have puppets that are anatomically correct (including internal organs) for children to play with and start IVs on. It's also easy to show a child how a gastric tube[1] will look on him or her or a broviac[2], or any number of various procedures. The child can take out the

---

1   Gastric tube: a surgically placed catheter that leads from the skin into the stomach. Liquid nourishment is poured into the catheter, which is capped on the skin's surface.

2   Broviac: a long term (2–6 years) indwelling catheter leading from the chest, through a vein into a chamber of the heart. Used for patients requiring frequent access to veins for medicine and blood draws. Reduces the need for painful pokes.

puppet's kidneys, give it a spica cast[3], and see what it looks like without its hair. Through play and manipulating medical objects such as blood pressure cuffs, syringes, and tourniquets, children can develop a sense of mastery over this terrifying place.

Child Life specialists also try to find out what a child's perception of his or her illness is, as well as perceptions of medical procedures. They try to help a child understand what's really going on. Once a little girl somberly told me, "I didn't know I had Kleenex under my skin." It took me a while, but then it dawned on me that someone had used the grown-up word "tissue," on this girl (i.e., "We're just going to take a little bit of tissue from underneath your skin to look at under the microscope.") Children are trying to make sense of the weird and frightening experience of hospitalization. They have fantastic imaginations that can distort or exaggerate information they receive about their illness. They also have the capacity to understand what is going on and why they are stuck in the hospital. The Child Life specialists help children through this realization in age appropriate ways. Other tools that are helpful include booklets filled with photos of a child's view of the operating room, computerized tomography (CT) scanner, magnetic resonance imaging (MRI), radiation, etc. Child Life specialists even change into scrubs to go down to the operating room with the child to provide a friendly face and reassurance until the child is sedated and asleep. When the child awakens in the recovery room, the Child Life specialist will be there, too.

Perfect place for a music therapist

Music therapy naturally complements the goals of Child Life. One of the most important things we can do for a hospitalized child is to normalize this alien environment with familiar music. We have the added benefit of an array of enticing instruments to offer a child who is terrified and distrustful of staff. Music is simply so different from the hospital experience –

---

3   Spica cast: A special cast for a younger child with a broken femur. Both legs are casted, with the cast running from the ankles to the hips, and a bar connecting the two legs. This does a better job of stabilizing the fracture and is supposed to be easier for the parents to manage.

it's fun, and it won't cause pain! A Child Life intern once told me, "You and the art therapist have such great toys! No wonder the kids want to play with you." It takes great toys to reach some of our patients.

Because normal life seems so far away when a child is hospitalized, it is crucial to recreate some sense of normalcy whenever we can. We stock the playroom with the accoutrements of childhood – modeling clay, paper, crayons, markers, paint, simple card games, board games, an array of puzzles, and lots of toys – to make this room look like home, preschool, daycare, or kindergarten. We get volunteers from the local universities to be available to play with kids. We have a foster grandparent program with seniors who hold babies and "fill in the gaps" for children when parents have to be at work.

Music is part of the normal experience of childhood. Little ones watch TV programs that are loaded with songs. As a music therapist on Pediatrics, it is my job to keep up with kids' songs. These are also songs of comfort that will feel familiar in this foreign environment. The playroom is a safe place where no exams or treatments or even taking medicine is allowed. The music therapy group, held in the playroom, is a place to make noise. It is the only time a kid can blow off some steam. And they do. Believe me when I say that asking a three-year-old boy to play the drum quietly is a lesson in futility. I have 35 rhythm instruments – shakers, scrapers, bells, rattles, and all sizes of drums. I have miniature shakers for tiny or very weak hands, bells that strap around a wrist or ankle, fat drumsticks for hands that can barely grasp, and really big drums that can stand up to intense banging. Any kid who is forced to undergo painful, invasive procedures is going to have a lot of energy and anger to vent. Banging on a drum is vastly preferable to banging on a nurse or parent. In fact, I have a rule in the music therapy group – if it didn't come out of my instrument bag, don't hit it with a stick. If they break, drums are replaceable.

There are children who are so emotionally traumatized by the process of hospitalization that they scream and hide under the bed covers whenever a staff member enters their room. This is not an uncommon response to the overwhelming rigors of hospitalization, and I've seen it in all age groups – toddler through teenager. A child like this will take some time to learn to trust staff. Whenever I'm referred to such a patient, I'll very quietly enter the room and introduce myself to the family. Then I'll sit near the bed and introduce myself to the patient. I'll tell him about the keyboard I brought with me. (I find keyboards to be nonthreatening and enticing – especially the one that has a motorcycle sound, or the recording keyboard you can burp into. A particularly interesting effect is created when I record some disgusting sound, i.e. a burp, and then play a well-known favorite song, *Twinkle Twinkle Little Star*, with the burp sound. There aren't many kids who can resist that combination.)

Because my patients may be so afraid of everyone coming through their door, I make myself as unthreatening as possible. I'll sit on low foot-stools, or on the floor to make myself appear smaller to the two-year-old sitting in a chair. I'll sit across the room from a wary, lonely toddler. I approach terrified children the same way I'd approach a frightened animal – quietly and slowly. I let the child determine our relationship. I offer my instruments, my humor, my friendship, and then leave it up to him to accept or refuse.

Empowering patients

Sometimes (and I cannot stress the importance of this enough) the most important thing I can do for my patients is to let them throw me out of the room. These children have very little control over their environment. Making choices is important for anyone's well-being, but for children it is especially important. A two-year-old is trying to gain mastery over her world – it's in her job description. But in being hospitalized, she may be forcibly returned to infantile dependency. Older kids who are used to a level of independence are forced to submit to any number of humiliating exams and painful procedures. These kids don't get a lot of opportunities to make their own decisions, so it is crucial that we set some up for them. And although they may want to, they can't throw the doctors or nurses out of the room.

How do you know when a child wants you out of the room? An older child will just say no to your offers. This needs to be respected. A younger child will let you know in subtle, nonverbal ways – screaming, crying, clutching onto mom for dear life, climbing the bars of the crib to get away from you, etc. Sometimes it's worth staying a little while to see if you can persuade them otherwise, but you never want to be the salesperson who sticks a foot in the door and refuses to leave. A therapeutic relationship won't develop from force. It has to be the child's call.

It's hard at first to feel honored when a child throws you out of the room; but we need to see it as a real step forward in that child's development and assertiveness. Most of the time the patient is so surprised that somebody actually listened to him and left, that the next time you come back, he'll be eager to interact with you. Once I met a nine-year-old girl in the Pediatric Intensive Care Unit who unfortunately had a lot of medical staff conferring among themselves in the corner of her room at the same time. She declined music therapy. On my way out of the unit, a nurse who wanted to refer another child to me stopped me in the hallway. While talking to the nurse (maybe two minutes), a doctor came up and said that now the girl wanted music therapy! This patient and I became very good friends over the course of her long stay and I believe it was because I let her throw me out of her room on our first interaction.

When a child throws you out, it's important to go back later, to keep offering music therapy. Eventually you'll start to look familiar to her and she'll be willing to give you a break. She'll also see you interacting with other kids in the playroom, or walking around the hallways armed with drums, guitar, or keyboards, and she'll be intrigued. But it's always important to give kids the choice of interacting with you or not.

Sometimes parents will decline your services for whatever reason. Most of the time it has nothing to do with you. It may be that they have just received overwhelming, terrible news regarding their infant and they cannot cope with another person at this time. Maybe the parents just had a fight and need to simmer down. It might also be due to the cycles of the moon, really bad food from the cafeteria, their least favorite nurse being on duty, or they feel a headache looming. The important thing is not to take rejection personally. I have had parents running after me, trying to explain why they don't want their child to have music today – they're afraid of hurting my feelings. I explain to them that my feelings are truly the least of their worries. I tell them it's OK to decline music therapy services. The last thing I want is to have parents worry about one more thing, especially on my account. Besides, another time the same parents will run after me, requesting that I sing to their child. It's important to offer the service and let the children or parents accept or decline.

Respect

Obviously it is important to respect the privacy of children and families when they are hospitalized. You always need to knock on a patient's door before barging in. However, you don't necessarily have to wait for an answer to quietly poke your head in. Many times I have been in a room with a teenager and heard someone knocking on the door. We both stop our conversation and look expectantly at the door, and most of the time the teenager remains silent. I've even asked, "Why don't you say, 'Come in'?" They just shrug. Unfortunately, I think people who are frequently hospitalized have given up on privacy long ago. So, if you knock and hear nothing from the other side, it may be that your patient is in the bathroom with the door closed and can't hear you, or your patient is new to this language and culture and is overwhelmed, or your patient has cerebral palsy and is nonverbal, or your patient is one of my silent teenagers and you could wait forever for an invitation to come in. It is considered polite to knock gently (there may be a sleeping baby in there with a sleep-deprived parent), and then quietly poke your head into the room. Also, be sure you're knocking on the real door to the patient's room, not the outer door of a double-doored isolation room, where you can knock all day and the only people who can hear you are the ones walking past you in the hallway.

Another issue of basic respect regards sitting on the child's bed. Thou shalt not sit on the bed of a patient without asking for permission from the child first. Not only may the child be in pain from your jostling the bed, it is considered a violation of his privacy. Asking for the child's permission will actually endear you to the patient because so few people treat children with that kind of respect.

Respect includes the way staff reacts to patients in coma, or even patients under the influence of sedating medications. Always assume your patient can hear you. Comatose patients, people hooked up to ventilators and heavily sedated, and kids on narcotics may look like they can't hear you, but many times they can. My internship supervisor had the experience of singing to a man in a coma who later was able to identify the songs the music therapist had sung to him. I recently listened to a teenager complain about his occupational therapist (OT). The patient had been on a narcotic for pain, and although he had been woozy, he'd heard and remembered everything the OT had said about him to her intern. They'd laughed at his attempts at speech, and had talked over him as if he were a car to repair. He did not appreciate this approach. In fact, it hardened his attitude toward his therapist and he became more resistant when she came to work with him on subsequent occasions.

One more thing: when working with one patient, quietly check out what his roommate is doing. Music therapy is rarely a silent activity (earphones being an exception), and most hospital rooms are not private. If I have a rambunctious patient with a sleeping roommate, I steer my high-energy child toward the playroom where we can make noise more freely.

Child development

Obviously it's a good idea to have a thorough understanding of child development if you're going to work in Pediatrics. If you have kids of your own, you probably have an even better understanding of child development. But keep in mind that the parameters of what's considered "normal" are very broad, and every child is unique. So even if you feel fairly confident on matters of child development, in working with hospitalized children you will see an even wider spectrum of normal development.

When working with little ones, it shouldn't take you too long to realize that you never want to get into a power play with a two-year-old. You'll never win. For example, I frequently see college volunteers trying to help me clean up after a music therapy group by wrestling a drumstick away from a toddler. A toddler's hand instinctively clamps down on an object whenever a grown-up attempts its retrieval. Since these kids already have to put up with an alarming amount of negative interactions from adults, we certainly don't want to create yet another problem for the child. And think about it – kids should be happy after our music group, not screaming!

Ideally we want to set up a situation where the young child can help us on his own volition. "Hey, Bobby – have you seen this cool car? Check it out! Vroom!" Bobby puts down my drumstick and picks up the car. Or, "Tessa, can you help me clean up this mess by putting all of the drumsticks into the big bag?" Preschoolers love all prepositions – in, out, over, under, etc. They love putting the instruments back into the bag. For those die-hard two-year-olds who absolutely have to take an instrument back to their rooms or they risk nuclear meltdown, I let them borrow the drum/shaker/stick. I know where they live (down the hall) and nothing I have is more important than a happy kid and parent. You may think I'm spoiling children. I am. But consider what these children are forced to endure and then tell me if this is the time or place to insist on perfect behavior. Cutting them a little slack while they're in the hospital does not create a monster.

Chronically ill kids face additional complications to normal development by virtue of dealing with pain and the inconvenience of hospitalization throughout their entire lives. They're also out of school a lot, and even if there's a school at the hospital, they're missing out on a lot of learning time due to illness. They're also missing out on their social contacts, which are very important. Children with chronic illness, such as sickle cell anemia, cystic fibrosis, and kidney disease are frequently smaller in stature compared to their peers.

One phenomenon of normal child development is that hospitalized children will usually be nicer to you than to their own families. This is because they realize you are not a person of pain, hopefully you are fun, and they want you to come back. So they will be on their best behavior for you in this strange new place. It is very common for a child to break down crying when her parent comes into the room. Newcomers to Pediatrics might assume the child prefers them to the parents, or may even suspect the parents of being abusive to their child. Nothing could be further from the truth. This is normal behavior. The child falls apart crying when the parent comes in because she is so desperate for that parent. She is overwhelmed with emotion. She knows she can be herself and her parent will still love her. Another interesting phenomenon of Pediatrics is that when the kids start to act sassy towards the staff, they are feeling much too healthy to be hospitalized and it's time for discharge.

Knowing appropriate parental behavior when you see it

Part of my job in the Child Life department is to advocate for children and model appropriate parenting behavior. One common problem we have is with parents who sneak out after their child has fallen asleep. It's the easy way out. It is hard to convince parents of the need to wake their child and tell her goodbye. But when the child awakens and finds no parent there, she panics and cries. This is a child who will soon resist sleep because she fears abandonment. It is amazing how long kids will refuse to fall asleep because of this fear. We tell the parents, "We would rather deal with the crying child after you tell her goodbye and leave, than deal with a child who doesn't trust adults."

One of my patients was a little boy who was hospitalized frequently for Hirschsprung's disease (a congenital intestinal disorder). He was about 16 months old. His well-meaning mom would bring him to the playroom, wait until he was engrossed in an activity, and then sneak off to take a shower. When he realized she was gone, he would fall apart. It got to the point that he cried hysterically if she brought him anywhere near the playroom because he knew she would ditch him there. This is not the response we want to engender in children when coming to the playroom.

Since I had a toddler at home at the time, I had recently attended a class on two-year-olds that was taught by a specialist from UC Davis Child Development Center. She told us that she still had abandonment issues because her parents would sneak out on her after she was asleep throughout her childhood. When I related this to the little boy's mom, we agreed to try a new approach. She would delay taking a shower until I arrived, and then I would be responsible for her son. The first day she said, "Danny, I'm going to take a shower. Kathy will take care of you until I get back. I'll only be gone a little while." She left, and of course he cried. The first day was the worst. He wouldn't distract to music or toys, so I carried him around the floor. I showed him where the shower was, and told him that mom would be out soon. We did the same thing over the next few days, each of which got a little easier for all of us. By the fourth day, Danny kissed mom goodbye and had no problems at all with her leaving him. During this process, Danny and I became best friends. His mom thought I was a miracle worker, but it was simple consistency and being honest with her son.

The job is five days/week

One thing we have all discovered within our Child Life department is the importance of being at the hospital every day. President Clinton had a famous sign in his office from his days as governor of Arkansas and during his first presidential campaign to keep him focused: "It's the economy, stupid." My favorite sign reads: "It's the relationship, stupid." Music therapy is frequently magical and often performs complete miracles, but it is only as therapeutic as the person offering the services. I have experienced both the weekly approach and the daily approach to the same Pediatric unit, and I have to say, daily is vastly superior. The weekly drop-in can be done, especially on Pediatrics where the kids are always ready for a good time. But daily contact is a completely different job, and so much more satisfying.

Both of my music therapy interns and the Child Life interns have borne this out as well. They also feel the need to be there five days/week. They'll say, "I'll just be getting close to a child on a Wednesday. How can I tell her, 'Bye – I'll see you next Monday?' It just doesn't work. You can't build a relationship on that."

Even with a daily job, you won't see the same child every day. There will be times when your patient is in surgery, or gone to scans or x-ray, or busy with a bunch of family or visitors, or just feeling too crummy to interact with you. But you'll see them often enough to build a very nurturing relationship that will help a child and family survive the rigors of hospitalization and illness. Although I only work halftime, I am there five days/week. Even then it can be hard to tell a child who is counting on me, "I'm going to be gone for a three-day weekend."

When I was on my first maternity leave, I saw the noted pediatrician, T. Berry Brazelton, on a news program. He stressed the importance of a consistent routine in a young child's life. He recommended that working moms set up the same schedule every day because it is far less disruptive for the baby/child. I have found that this approach is also the best for my patients. They have so little that is normal or consistent in their hospital stay. Their nurses are there for a few days, then off for several. Kids are constantly being whisked off for x-rays and scans. "Hurry up and wait," seems like the institutional mantra. If consistency is important with healthy kids, it is exponentially more important to be consistent with kids who are ill and stuck in a hospital.

Therefore, our music therapy group occurs Monday through Friday at 11:30 am. All the nurses know about the music therapy group. In fact, it is the only playroom activity that does occur every day. The music therapy group is so important to the kids and nurses (and especially to me) that we try to schedule as much as we can around it. The rehabilitation team (physical therapy, occupational therapy, speech pathology) is great about scheduling their twice-daily treatments around music therapy group if their patient is appropriate for it. If a child has to miss our group one day because of surgery, or x-ray, or just because he's feeling punk, I can say, "Don't worry, we have music therapy group every day." I love to say that. It almost makes the day sound normal.

3. The Group Experience

Music therapy group

Music in a group is a place where magic can happen on a daily basis. It is truly a situation where the whole is greater than the sum of its parts. A group of strangers comes into the playroom, everyone picks up a drum and somehow a sense of community is born. The amount of energy and sheer fun that can occur constantly amazes me. Music therapy group is my favorite part of the day. There are kids and even volunteers who think it's the only thing I do all day. (I honestly work with a lot of kids at the bedside, too.)

I told my interns, "You can do anything in the music therapy group but be boring." If you're boring, no one will come back. A litmus test is: If you're bored, chances are very good that your group is bored, too. Boredom is not an option. These kids and families are stuck in a hospital, for heaven's sake! They're not picky about entertainment. It's you or TV or video games. And if you're real exciting, they'll even choose you over video games. That's a real honor. (Of course, they may just be bored from having spent the previous 24 hours straight playing the video game, but still I'm honored.)

So, you owe these people a good time. This is not hard to do, but first you've got to convince them to come. I get various responses when I invite folks to the music therapy group. New patients don't want to come without their parents, and parents can be reticent to come, thinking I might ask them to perform a solo rendition of *Oh Holy Night*. They'll say,

"Oh, I can't sing!" I then tell them my motto – If you can't sing well, sing loud. I come from a family of loud singers. Absolutely no one in my group is intimidated by my vocal abilities – in fact, they feel encouraged to join in if only to drown me out.

On two separate occasions now, visitors who have been given a tour of Pediatrics during music therapy group have asked in all earnestness, "Is construction going on?" When I heard that, I considered going out and buying us all hard hats. Truly we are not as loud as a bunch of pile drivers, although I have a collection of earplugs that have all proven ineffective. I know it will be a miracle if I enter my golden years with my hearing intact, but I can't hear myself sing with ear plugs in – and these people are already suffering enough without me guessing at the pitch.

Sometimes I find people who are afraid of drums of any kind – even afraid of noise of any kind. I do allow kids to make noise in our music group. We have a door – luckily one of those substantial fire doors – that we can close when we get a little loud. But I believe that kids (and adults) have a primal need to vent energy and emotions, and my music therapy group is just about the only place they can do that in the hospital setting.

In college I took a percussion class. Whenever I was frustrated over some other class, I'd go practice drums. I felt the exhilaration of pounding out my frustrations while making a beautiful sound on the timpani, or creating thunder from a drum roll on the bass drum. The snare, of course, required too much concentration, but the big drums were truly primal therapy. I extend that opportunity to the kids and parents in my music therapy group. I tell shy parents, "This is your chance to play drums! How often do you get an invitation like that?" Every once in a while, we get a parent who played drums in high school and we all have a great time. I've also had some children who were simply born to play drums – they were truly gifted. Music therapy group is always a good time.

Sometimes when I invite a patient to music therapy group, the parents are very supportive of their child going, but they roll their eyes at me, suggesting that maybe the group is a little too musical for them. I tell these parents, "I serve Tylenol chasers."

Safety first – group instruments

There are three requirements for pediatric instruments:

1. They must be safe.

2. They must be able to be cleaned with a germicide.

3. They must stand up to abuse.

In picking instruments I ask myself – What can a toddler do to this? Is it slobber-proof? Is it small enough to disappear inside a mouth? (We've had some wide-mouthed babies.) Can a child's razor sharp teeth separate the bell from the plastic wristband, or the bead from the string? I remove all the small rubber heads from my drumsticks and reattach them with superglue, but I still wouldn't bet a child's life on them. Many has been the time when a college volunteer has held a little one on her lap with both of them facing into the music therapy group. The child is happily gnawing on the rubber ball of the drumstick but the volunteer can only see the back of the child's head. This always happens when I'm leading a song and I try to communicate the sense of imminent danger to the volunteer by facial tic, shaking my head, and general look of alarm. Most of the time I have to stop the group and hand a more appropriate shaker to the child. My goal is to avoid ending up on the evening news: "Music therapy group kills child at the Medical Center. Film at 11:00!"

Maracas from Mexico are inexpensive and colorful, but I'm sure there must be lead in the paint. Don't hand these to any child who will ulti-mately stick them into his mouth. It's handy to have a stash of nearly edible (good to teethe on) instruments that will not break apart and are easily hosed down for toddlers.

I have cabinets with key locks in the playroom for my instruments. I compulsively relock them after I take an instrument out because if I don't, I know that as soon as I turn my back a toddler will wander over there, pull out a keyboard or drum, and drop it onto his head. Again, I want to avoid, "Film at 11:00!"

It's hard to comprehend just how quickly toddlers can act. One of my fieldwork situations in college was with deaf preschoolers. I remember a session where we were all sitting on the floor. I set my guitar down in front of me while I turned around to get something else. I turned my back on a half-dozen three-year-olds for maybe 30 seconds and when I faced forward again, out of the corner of my eye I saw them all pulling their hands back quickly into their laps. They were wide-eyed and smiling and I thought, hmm... But I didn't know what they had done until I strummed my guitar. That's right. A preschooler simply can't resist those little white tuning pegs. My guitar sounded like it had been tuned by Schoenberg, himself, after a night of binge drinking. I was forever impressed by the speed of little ones.

Be aware that a toddler will grab onto any dangling strap and pull on it, thereby pulling a drum off the table and onto her head. This tendency is the horrible and frequent cause of burns in toddlers – the dangling cord of the coffee pot that must be yanked. It's difficult, but you must anticipate what children will do because they are much faster than you. There is no way you can move quickly enough to stop some dangerous action once they've started it unless you're sitting right next to them.

So what will they do? Babies will stick everything into their mouths. Don't get into a power play with them, saying, "No, no, don't put that in your mouth!" Just give them a small but sturdy plastic maraca that they can chew on. Toddlers and preschoolers are very dexterous and have a physiological need to poke, turn, twist, unscrew, nudge, pull, push, and pry. They will perform all of these maneuvers quite deftly on all of your instruments. Your job is to steer them towards safe ones. Also make sure they have plenty of room during music therapy group so that they don't poke their drumsticks into the face of their neighbor accidentally or not so accidentally. Educate your volunteers and peripheral staff members who may be helping you with the group on how to keep the kids safe. And politely model appropriate behavior for parents – "This rubber maraca might be better for your baby to gnaw on than that goat hoof shaker."

Predictably instruments fall over, and fall off the table with alarming frequency during music therapy groups. Keep big drums on the floor so they won't have as far to fall, and hopefully won't take out a child in the process. Things fall so often, in fact, that I have begun to look on it as a sort of litmus test for my drums. Does this instrument sound as good falling off the table as when we're playing it? Different drums fall better than others. My 16-year-old barrel conga falls like a judo expert. Its rounded sides spread the shock throughout the drum and it rolls just beautifully. By contrast, I'm amazed that my new straight-sided conga is still in one piece. It makes a horrifying sound when it goes over. When you're shopping for instruments, surreptitiously drop them on a hard surface and watch and listen for your best buys. Of course, you'll probably be asked to leave several music stores, so use discretion.

Parents in the group

Parental behavior in the music therapy group is always interesting to observe. The group is the perfect opportunity for parents and children (patient and siblings) to act together as a family again in a fairly normal way. Singing favorite songs, being silly together, laughing – putting the stress on the back burner for a while – is absolutely essential in this environment. Parental roles get tweaked during hospitalization. Many times parents aren't sure where their caretaker roles end and the nurse's begins. Parents are sometimes called upon to hold their child for a painful procedure. In fact, some children prefer that their parent hold them rather than a nurse. Then there are children who feel they are being hospitalized because of their naughty behavior. There is nothing more heartbreaking than to hear a child tell his parents, "I'm sorry! Please take me home! I promise I'll be good!" We've got to offer some opportunity for normal family life here.

Once I met a mom in the hallway near the elevator. She was suffering the pain and helplessness of watching her child as he lay sedated and attached to a ventilator in the Pediatric Intensive Care Unit. I told her what I did as a music therapist and invited her to the 11:30 group. She came. She needed to see some semblance of normal childhood. She needed help in believing that her child would eventually be one of the members of the music therapy group. She came daily to the group and drummed, and sang, and helped out with the other children. It was a wonderful day when her son was finally able to join us in the group.

There are times, particularly when a child is newly diagnosed with some dreadful disease, when both mother and child come to music therapy group and share a chair. The patient, who is still feeling fairly well, participates quietly from the safety of mom's lap, while his mother cries softly behind her child. In these situations, I feel both their needs are being met.

Immigrant families can have a great time in the music therapy group. Drums are universal. They have social, religious, and even medicinal significance in many cultures. For a family who is trying to adjust to a new language and culture to have to make the additional adjustment to a hospital may be overwhelming. Western medicine's views on disease are completely different from the way illness is perceived in the mountains of Southeast Asia. However, when these families unite in the playroom over drums, we are all the same. For the first time, I'll see the parents smile as they pick up a drum and look it over. Drums bridge the gap.

Years ago we had a Sikh family from India. The mother brought her three-year-old son to every music therapy group during the course of his hospitalizations for leukemia. She loved an instrument I'd made out of wood and bottle caps during my impoverished student days (I call it the Dr Pepper shaker). She said it sounded just like an instrument they used in India during sacred ceremonies and reminded her of home. She played it exclusively whenever they attended music therapy group.

Group songs

I choose songs for the group based on familiarity to children. These are the songs they sing in preschool and kindergarten, and that appear on various children's TV shows. The exception is *Sesame Street*. Although *Sesame Street* is my favorite show on television, their songs are truly brilliant, and therefore beyond my feeble abilities on guitar. They are also not terribly singable for the average preschooler (lucky for me). We frequently play a CD of *Sesame Street* favorites in the playroom as background music during other activities. However, although the playroom assistant and I love to sing along to these, the kids don't seem to.

When the songs are familiar to most of the kids, my groups tend to be more successful. An exception to this is if a new song is simple enough and repetitious – then it can easily be taught to the group. And if we can incorporate the new song into the group on the following day, with a lot of the same kids – presto – we'll have another familiar song for the group. Remember, this is a large Pediatric unit – we have lots of chronically ill children who will be returning to the hospital and to the music therapy group.

For the most part however, the group is not the setting to do new songs. There is so much in the hospital environment that is absolutely alien that offering children a familiar song is throwing them a lifeline. Another exception to the "familiar is superior" rule, though, is when we have a big, noisy group that needs to bang long and hard on the drums, and it really doesn't matter what I sing because they're not going to hear me anyway! If that's the case, I pick a long song with a driving rhythm that will just let them play until they're worn out (e.g. *She'll Be Coming 'Round the Mountain*). It's the equivalent of running an Irish setter behind your car to exhaust that endless energy. (This is a metaphor – please do not run your dog, or your children, behind your car!)

I like to put the word "love" into a song wherever I can. If I'm singing a farm song and using every toy the child has in the crib for a visual aid, I'll grab the teddy bear and give it a sound: "I love you." I'll also have the bear kiss the child simultaneously. It can be a bit of a tongue twister, but I just slow down the rhythm and make it work. I don't mind singing the *Barney* song (lyrics by Lee Bernstein) because my philosophy is you just can't have enough love when you're a kid stuck in the hospital.

Kids like to teach me their favorite songs, which can be a real challenge. Most children are not members of the Vienna Boys' Choir – they have not yet developed a reliable sense of pitch or melody – so it's a bit of a stretch to get a song from a child in its real version. Speaking of pitch, I know the literature shows that children's voices are higher than adults, which implies that music therapists should pitch songs higher when working with them. And if you are, indeed, a bass perhaps you could sing in falsetto. But if you are not naturally a soprano or tenor, don't sweat it. If you're squeaking or straining during the music therapy group, it's going to be far more painful for everyone in your group than if you were just singing in a range comfortable for you. Keep in mind that all of their parents who are singing in the group with you will have lower voices and will also be squeaking and straining. The kids will be happy singing in whatever range is comfortable for you, and your voice will last years longer.

It should come as no surprise that we frequently get silly on songs. We change lyrics around to include love, but also to be ridiculous. Kids and families are desperate for an opportunity to laugh in this setting (as well as doctors and nurses). Blowing off steam, anger, frustration, and energy by banging on a drum and singing together are indispensable. When the kids are happy, the parents are happy. The nurses come into the playroom and see the families in a different light and they're happy. Music therapy group is so much fun for everyone, how could it possibly be boring?

Here are some of the absolute favorite songs for my music therapy group these days.

The Wheels on the Bus (traditional)

This has been a standard for years, and I sing it so often that one family actually gave me a little wooden school bus pin to put onto my name badge. We've changed it around a little – instead of the mommies saying, "Shhh", we have the mommies and daddies saying, "I love you." Again, my personal belief is that there are plenty of people in a hospital telling children "Shhh" and not enough saying, "I love you." We also added a verse at the end in my honor. I commute daily by bus and this verse is the story of my life. It goes, "The people at the stop yell, 'Hold that bus!'"

Bingo (was his name-o) (traditional)

Probably the oldest song in my repertoire. I explain *BINGO* each time we sing it to the kids because I remember being chronically confused in the first grade while the rest of the class sang *BINGO*. Suddenly one day the heavens opened up and a light came down upon my head, and I finally understood what was going on! "Hey! Now I get it! They're dropping a letter every time! I finally get *BINGO!*" So, for all those six-year-olds like me who just don't get it, I explain: "This time we're not going to say the letter B – we'll just bang on the drum, instead, like this." Then, "OK, this time no Bs or Is, we're just going to call this poor dog, 'NGO.'"

Down by the Bay (traditional)

Currently my favorite group song. This is a very popular rhyming song that is great for ages five and up. Lots of kids are currently exposed to this song in kindergarten, although not all of them catch on to rhymes at that early an age. Even though they're not ready to create their own rhymes, they enjoy memorizing the short verses in the song. Older kids can get very creative in inventing long and elaborate rhymes, i.e., "Have you ever seen a whale with a polka-dot tail, reading his mail, while going to jail, for eating a snail, in a giant pink pail?" Or, my personal favorite, "Have you ever seen a dragon who was always braggin' about his little red wagon? His tail was waggin', but his belly was saggin'!" This is also a good exercise for older music therapists like myself who are trying to keep our memories intact and dementia at bay!

Five Little Ducks (traditional)

This is a basic countdown song that can be adapted to lots of favorite animals, i.e. cats, dogs – we recently did worms (instead of "quack", they "wiggled"). I actually went to a concert of "Trout Fishing in America" (one of my favorite groups) and they abused the audience with this song. They made us start at "99 Little Ducks", and if we didn't quack loud enough, they raised the number!

Six Little Ducks (traditional)

This is the song to sing when you feel the need to quack. Lots of quacking in this song – you really get your money's worth. It's a good choice when you have little ones who may not be verbal, or speak English, but love animal noises. Hand gestures are an easy accompaniment.

Five Little Freckled Frogs (Wood and Scott 1954)

This moves right along with a driving beat in case you need a long, fast moving, run-out-their-energy type of song.

Five Little Monkeys (jumping on the bed) (traditional)

This is a big crowd-pleaser. Kids seem to appreciate the idea of monkeys jumping on the bed. Go figure.

I Like to Eat Apples and Bananas (traditional)

This is a good song for kids who understand the different vowel sounds (five years and up). I recently heard of a new way to sing it – substitute "pepperoni pizza" for the apples and bananas! ("I like to ate, ate, ate paperoni paza!" This takes practice! The first time I sang it, my brain hurt from the concentration!)

Itsy Bitsy Spider (traditional)

This is a truly beloved song of the infant and preschooler set. They enjoy the hand motions, even though they get stuck on putting both their thumbs together, and their index fingers together, and then can't figure out why their fingers don't go anywhere. (You must have a thumb touching an index finger to be successful – I discovered this at age 18.) The only problem with the spider song is that it's too short. We experimented around with different options for many years – singing it twice, writing new verses (that nobody knew). Then the movie *Spiderman* came out and solved my problem perfectly. Now we do a second verse with Spidey!

> *Itsy Bitsy Spiderman went up the waterspout*
> *Down came the rain and washed poor Spiderman out!*
> *Out came the sun and dried up all the rain*
> *And Itsy Bitsy Spiderman went up the spout again.*

Of course, the hand motions change from tiny fingers to miming whole hands going up the window in more of a suction cup manner. Our playroom assistant loves this verse and tends to make hand motions more in keeping with a flash flood when Spiderman gets washed out. The rest of the hand motions are the same.

Old MacDonald (traditional)
The kids will also refer to this song as "E-I-E-I-O." Although it is another good one for jogging my memory when I include every child's animal in the group on every rendition, in the interest of time I frequently drop the repeats.

Down on Grandpa's Farm (traditional)
This is a great song for various ages. Little kids love to make the animal sounds, and older kids get fantastically silly on it. For example, when asked, "What is your favorite animal?" a ten-year-old may say, "I want a purple polka-dotted cow who says, 'Quack.'" It's a little confusing for the three-year-olds, but it's endlessly hilarious for the older kids. And since older kids add a lot of fun to music therapy groups, we want to keep them happy.

Do Your Ears Hang Low? (traditional)
For this song you must have volunteers who are willing to appear a bit foolish. Our volunteers are almost all college students who are usually

motivated by the following phrase: "You will get an 'A' if you do this." The hand gestures are fairly easy, but the song repeats over and over, gaining in acceleration on each repetition. As the volunteers' hands are flying, they run the risk of slapping themselves or the person next to them, which is a hazard but also entertaining for the rest of us! Our playroom assistant and I are always in keen competition during this song. By the last and fastest repetition I just slur all the words together and play the guitar as fast as I possibly can. I usually beat her but, of course, that is my perspective.

If All the Raindrops Were Lemon Drops & Gumdrops (traditional)

This is also known as the "sticking out your tongue song." My three-year-old niece taught it to me many years ago. It's a song about the weather – if the raindrops and snowflakes were candy, we'd be out there catching them in our teeth! It allows kids to do something socially unacceptable (sticking out your tongue) in a fun and acceptable manner. It's also a valuable song for little ones working on speech, and kids recovering from head injuries where they really need to practice moving their tongues.

Twinkle Twinkle Little Star / ABC Song (traditional)

There are many adults who don't realize that this is the same melody for two different songs. These are absolute favorite songs for many little ones – songs of comfort and home. The alphabet song is also great for immigrant children learning English. I have been so touched to see every adult in the room – parents to pre-med college volunteers – singing the alphabet song together during our music groups.

She'll Be Coming 'Round the Mountain (traditional)

This is a truly great old standard. Everybody knows it, or else should learn it. It has fun hand motions, a driving beat, and you can substitute favorite foods (pepperoni pizza fits in perfectly for chicken and dumplings) and favorite colors (for pajamas) to personalize it. It also provides a wonderful background for rewriting with your own verses.

> Oh we'll have to take out the garbage
> When she comes – P U! (gesture: hold your nose)

Where is Thumbkin? (traditional)
Another preschool favorite, this is a hand gesture song that I sing without using the guitar – the fingers are that important. I recently learned Spanish lyrics that go with this melody.

> *Buenos dias, buenos dias,*
> *¿Como estas? ¿Como estas?*
> *Muy bien, gracias, muy bien, gracias,*
> *¿Y Usted? ¿Y Usted?*

So get some books on children's songs and build your own repertoire. Be sure to include slow, quiet songs for lullabies at the bedside/crib side, and fast, driving songs for big groups with lots of energy. Like any other activity in music therapy, keep track of which songs work, and which songs don't. Also be advised that there will be regional differences in songs. Kids from Oregon sometimes know different words to *The Wheels on the Bus* than California kids. And what's very interesting is that animals in other countries make different sounds from American animals! I discovered this one day when I walked out into the rain with a Danish friend. I said, "This is great weather for ducks." She made a funny noise and I asked, "Why are you making a frog sound?" She said, "I'm not. I'm making a duck sound." Apparently ducks in Denmark sound a lot like American frogs. We went through the entire repertoire of animal noises and found other discrepancies. I have since found that Mexican animals have different noises as well. This is endlessly fascinating for me. Someday I'll get a grant to go around the world and collect preschool impersonations of animal noises. Won't that be a fun book? Meanwhile, back to the group.

Cue the group

I give a lot of visual cues during our songs, using my hands and body to help kids along. This helps little ones in my groups, as well as kids with head injuries, and folks whose first language is not English.

Using my body for cues becomes more critical for bigger groups. Our daily music therapy group ranges from very small to very large. Sometimes we'll have a group that consists of one kid, two parents, two volunteers, and me (the group of one, I call it; or how many grown-ups does it take to run a music therapy group?). Ironically, if I have a huge group, every volunteer will call in sick that day. Our groups have also been standing room only, with patients, parents, siblings, cousins, sometimes a kid in bed in traction, friends, and periodically, it seems, a patient's entire daycare on a field trip to visit the hospital! These groups can be so noisy that I can't even hear myself sing (though I can feel my lips move) and I certainly can't hear my guitar. On these occasions I stand and exaggerate my strumming so that the folks in the back of the room don't speed up and pass those of us in the front. Sometimes I bob up and down to the beat and search every grown-up in the back for eye contact so that they understand where we are. I have a really big mouth, and grew up in a large family, so I can project.

I've met several music therapists who prefer to dwell in the land of quiet. I really don't know what they would do in these situations. I know in theory it's very possible to be a quiet music therapist. I just don't know how.

Adults in the music therapy group will not only drive and speed up your group; they're also uncomfortable with silence. If you ask a child for a favorite animal for a farm song and that child takes more than three seconds to come up with an answer, the adults will jump in and make suggestions – "Do you like dogs? Cats? Horses? Pigs? Armadillos?" They can overwhelm the child. You need to delicately redirect the question back to the child, lean in closely and try to get his answer.

Speaking of armadillos, periodically kids have given me a farm full of their favorite mute animals: rabbits, flamingoes, giraffes, rhinos, and lizards. This is a chance to get creative. What sound does the animal make when it moves? When it eats? Hop, crunch, slither, and sticking out your tongue in lizard fashion are all appropriate responses here. Or, if absolutely nothing comes to mind, ask, "So, Bobby, what's your second favorite animal?"

Changing the group to fit individual needs

It is important to feel the mood of the group while leading it, and to change the tempo of the songs if need be. Maybe we'll have a child from the rehabilitation service who needs extra time to get the words out. Sometimes it's been effective for the speech pathologist to join us to give one-to-one attention to a patient during the fun experience of music therapy group.

Children who are new to the hospital and therefore new to the group may be understandably nervous – especially if their first group is rambunctious. You really can't tell how a child will do in their first group. I've seen kids stare wide-eyed at the other kids. I've had little ones cry in the downtime between songs. As soon as we start singing again, they stop crying. That tells me to have very little downtime in that group. Don't talk – just keep singing! Some children cry if you give them eye contact – I call them the "Don't look at me" kids. So I don't.

A recurring phenomenon is the number of babies who fall asleep in the music therapy group. It seems the louder the group is – the more babies fall asleep. In fact, when I'm rounding up my usual suspects for music therapy group and I see a frantic parent trying to get a tired but resisting baby down for a nap, I'll tell them, "If your baby won't go to sleep, bring her to music therapy group. Somehow babies fall asleep in the group." My own theory is that babies trust noise and they trust other kids. They finally let down their guard in the group setting and sleep overtakes them. Then again, maybe the group qualifies as "white noise" – like the vacuum cleaner! Or construction!

There are times when I'm returning to the playroom from rounding up kids for group and from down the hallway I hear the kids pounding on the tables, in prison riot fashion, chanting, "We want music! We want music!" This gives me a warm, tingly and just a teensy bit of an apprehensive feeling – I wonder how loud this group is going to be! Still, there is nothing like the daily music therapy group.

Drum improvisation group

There are times when the majority of my group population is comprised of older kids. They may or may not want to sing songs together. This is the perfect time for a drum improvisation group. Everyone chooses a drum (it helps to have a healthy assortment of big drums – congas, djembes, etc. – because regardless of what they say, kids know that size does matter and everyone wants a big drum). We all take turns being the leader, with the rest of the group trying to follow the demonstrated rhythm. This can be an amazing experience. When the group is in sync, it feels good down to your toes. You can actually feel the music flowing through the group and through your own body! Of course, when the group is having difficulty following the leader, it is chaotic through and through, too. Drum groups have an element of magic to them.

Hussy!

Sometimes I need to work with a new patient on a one-to-one basis because he is restricted to bed, or too tired or sick to come to music therapy group. We develop a relationship based on these private sessions, and then as the child feels better he comes to the playroom and group. This can be where some interesting dynamics kick into play. The child, who is used to my undivided attention, is suddenly sharing me with a room full of other kids. The very idea that I see children other than him can be very difficult to accept, and suddenly I realize what the child is thinking – "You hussy!"

I actually had a three-year-old boy climb onto the table in front of me, and cup my face in his hands during the middle of music therapy group to get my attention. I remember thinking – "Maybe Eric is not such a group player!" It's funny, but it's also a bit of a problem. It's a delicate balance to attend to each child in the group. You have to be sure you give your old-timers the attention they're used to, and at the same time make the new kids feel welcome and secure. I think of the group as similar to having 20 plates spinning on long, slender poles, and I have to keep all of them from crashing to the ground.

4. The Importance
of Being
Staff

Recognizing the expertise of others

Sometimes music therapists think we can do it all, but it is essential to respect the expertise of other disciplines and to work together as a team. Although I can certainly aim individual sessions and groups to complement the goals of physical therapy, occupational therapy, speech therapy and even respiratory therapy, my job is primarily one of providing support and fun to my patients. If there is specific information I need to know, I will stop the physical therapist (PT) or occupational therapist (OT) in the hallway and ask them, "Show me how far you want Brandon to move his arm." During the pediatric rehabilitation team meetings is a great time to gather this type of information. Once the therapists know you're interested in complementing their goals, they'll poke their heads into the playroom to update you. These exchanges take only moments, but they are invaluable. You can also read the chart, but oftentimes they'll write something like, "Patient able to abduct right trapezius to 30 degrees." And I always seem to have left my protractor at home. The important thing is to ask.

Finding out what the physical limitations are for a patient is critical for our volunteers and playroom staff as well. We never want to put our patients in a dangerous position or hurt them in any way. Likewise, I am never going to stretch my patients in painful range of motion (ROM) exercises. That's not my job. But I do need to know if I should gently encourage my ten-year-old patient who has recently become an incomplete quadriplegic to use the gross motor action of her left arm as well as her stronger right arm to play the keyboard.

One year we had two children admitted to the hospital over the course of a few months. Both had cerebral palsy, both were in special education classes, and both had broken femurs because their teachers had done ROM exercises on them! Their teachers broke their legs! Needless to say, their parents were quite displeased with these teachers. And everyone wondered why special education teachers were performing ROM exercises on these kids anyway. After all, the children were already being seen by a slew of therapists who were just a bit more qualified in that arena.

The medical dictum, "Do no harm," is applicable here. A music therapist on Pediatrics is a support person for the child and the family. We do not hold patients down for nursing or medical procedures, and we do not stretch patients in painful exercises. But we do provide support wherever we can. Additionally we can provide an opportunity where a child would be willing to push himself in a fun environment.

Co-treating

I came upon a three-year-old patient of mine in the Burn Unit one day who was walking for the first time with the PT. This child, who just the day before had been laughing and singing with me, was now screaming in pain. I said, "I think we need a marching song!" I grabbed my guitar from my shoulder and started singing, *The Ants Go Marching* (traditional), and this little boy fell right into step. He stopped screaming and walked the entire length of the unit with his PT. At the end of the hall we ran out of song, and the child resumed screaming. The PT looked up at me and frantically said, "Sing another song!" The music provided distraction, focus, and rhythm for this child, as well as something familiar and enjoyable.

I hold patients' hands and encourage them to do deep breathing exercises while they're being stretched by physical therapy or occupational therapy. I tell them jokes. I sing songs. And as soon as the therapists are gone, I make sure we do something fun. Something good always has to follow something bad.

One time I was working with a great little five-year-old boy on keyboards. He moaned when the PT walked in. (They get that a lot – they have a tough job.) I suggested that we do his exercises to the keyboard music. He leapt at the idea, picked a great rhythm and proceeded to lead all of us – his mom, the PT and me – in a workout Jane Fonda would've been proud of. He had control over three grown-ups, and was getting his exercises done in a fun way with a huge smile on his face. Even the PT was smiling.

The PTs and OTs are very sensitive and hesitant to infringe on my relationships with the children. It helps them in their work when I'm available to co-treat, but I don't want the child to begin to associate me with painful procedures. This becomes a problem with the Child Life specialists, too. The child sees the specialist coming in with a backpack full of distracting toys and knows that an unpleasant procedure is just around the corner. You are a support person – not someone the kids should dread! It is critical to have additional, positive therapy time with the patient if you are going to co-treat during painful procedures. Another approach is to invite the Child Life specialists, PTs and OTs in to join you and the child during a music therapy group or individual session. That way the child has a chance to have fun with these other professionals in a different, and more enjoyable, setting.

In music therapy group we can promote treatment goals in a fun environment. Whereas a child will yell in pain during occupational therapy, that same child will get a similar workout banging on a drum in the music therapy group. Once I was with a six-year-old boy who was suffering from neuropathy. This was an unfortunate side effect of his chemotherapy that left his arms and legs severely weakened and in a lot of pain. The neurology team came into his room to examine him. He screamed when they moved his arms to measure passive ROM. As soon as they walked out the door, I handed this boy a drum and a mallet. He swung his arms in a much wider arc to bang on the drum, laughing the whole time. I looked at his dad and asked, "Should we call those doctors back in?" Kids will do things in music therapy of their own volition and happily because they are in control and they're having fun.

It amazed me to watch one of my nine-year-old patients in the music therapy group. He was a wonderful guy, well known to us because of his sickle cell anemia. He'd suffered a cerebral vascular accident (CVA) and was undergoing extensive inpatient rehabilitation. He'd always been a musical kid before his stroke, and now in the music therapy group he was able to coordinate many parts of his body – tapping his foot to the beat, playing a rhythm on the drum, bobbing his torso up and down, and singing a song – all at the same time. A combination of bodily movements that would have required too much concentration under other circumstances was attained effortlessly while he was swept up in the music and the process of having a good time.

Celebrations

We celebrate lots of events on Pediatrics. Most of the staff dresses in costume for Halloween. We also outfit the kids with costumes and make-up and have a party catered by the cafeteria with punch and cookies. We are lucky enough to have a very generous community that donates costumes and toys to our department, so we have a ready stash of presents. Kids who have to spend a birthday in the hospital get a wrapped present, a small cake/large cupcake from the cafeteria, and of course, the staff singing *Happy Birthday* (Hill and Hill 1934). The oncology kids get a party for the end of chemotherapy. (Although they may be returning to the clinic for outpatient chemo for the next several months, at least they won't have to be hospitalized.) We celebrate the discharge day for the inpatient rehabilitation kids. And, of course, we have a song for every occasion.

In writing my party songs, I adhere to the KISS principle (Keep It Simple, Stupid). All of the words are sung to the tunes of two well-known songs – *For He's a Jolly Good Fellow*, or *She'll Be Coming 'Round the Mountain* (both traditional). Everybody knows these tunes, and my lyrics repeat a lot. I can meet with a crowd of staff members in the hallway and go over the song quickly, then take the group into a room to sing and we're great.

It helps if the songs are funny. For instance, my end of inpatient chemo song is:

> *For this is your last in-house chemo,*
> *For this is your last in-house chemo,*
> *For this is your last in-house chemo,*
> *The rest are all out-house.*

Now, when we sing this song to a three-year-old, the child will smile at us and wonder why her mother is laughing so hard. I think one of the reasons I never have a problem finding nurses who are willing at a moment's notice to come into a room and sing with me is because my songs are easy to learn and silly. One nurse did tell me, however, "You know, Kathy, I just get a picture of hanging chemotherapy in an outhouse and I have to tell you, something just gets to me a little." Nurses have a cleanliness fixation.

This next information is basic, but why should you have to make the same mistakes I've made? If you are the only one with a guitar in a group of people, you'd think they'd look to you for the starting pitch. Well, *only if you've trained them!* In many situations, my singers have taken off with the song before I even had my guitar strapped on. That's when we get a rendition of *Happy Birthday* (Hill and Hill 1934) in six different keys with four different rhythms. Look, the kid has enough trouble just being in the hospital, let's not make this harder on the family! While I'm out in the hallway teaching the song to my staff singers, I'll tell them, "Watch me!" This is very important. You may have spent your life in the choir, but the nurses haven't. Then inside the room I'll tell the child how proud we all are of him, Child Life will hand over the present, I'll strum a chord, hum the pitch and get everybody's eye, then we're off! That way we sound great, and we all have a good time.

One day I came back from vacation and was stopped by several reha-bilitation (rehab) therapists throughout the day. They begged me to either never go on vacation again, or to make a tape of the rehab discharge song for the times when I was not available to help them sing it. Apparently they'd tried to sing the song without me and had rather disastrous results. Once you get used to sounding fairly good, it's hard to go back to lousy – it's just too embarrassing. It's not as if my hospital is loaded with great singers, but there is more than enough love, support and energy to make up for what we lack in vocal expertise.

Nurse as ally

On our floor we practice family-centered care. We encourage parents to continue their role of primary caretakers for their children – to hold, feed, change diapers, bathe – as much as possible within the parameters of the disease or injury. The nurses show the parents how to safely manage the caretaking duties and are always available to help out, but nothing is more therapeutic for the child than having a parent close by. We have sleep chairs next to every bed and encourage parents to spend the night whenever they can. I have seen kids who were at death's door, who by all rights should have died, but survived because their parents refused to leave them. The power of parental love is something to behold.

It is also important for the child to retain his place in the family. In chronically ill kids, this becomes a real problem. Anytime the child is hospitalized, the family grows accustomed to getting along without him. The child knows that, and resents the fact that his siblings are still included in the family while he's stuck in the hospital in terrible pain. We're trying to hold families together here. We're also trying to get these kids back to their normal lives as soon as we can – to avoid the feeling of becoming institutionalized.

Our nursing staff also practices primary nursing. Any child admitted to the hospital is assigned to a specific team of nurses. During this and any future stays, the family will always belong to this team. Within the team, a few nurses will agree to be that child's primary nurse. This means that whenever that nurse is available, she or he will work with that family. This leads to nurses who really know their patients, and families who know and trust their nurses.

In other areas of the hospital I've run into situations where a child has been in for a month, and it seems he's never gotten the same nurse twice. This means that the parent is constantly explaining basics to the new nurse – there's a lot of reinventing the wheel. This is wasted expertise. Primary nurses know everything about their patients and often grow deeply bonded to their families. These nurses are a wonderful resource for a music therapist.

I rely on our nursing staff tremendously. They know which kids are withdrawn or have no families at the bedside. They know which families are going to receive very bad news that day and try to arrange to have someone from our department available to play with the child and/or the siblings while the parents talk with the doctors. The nurses will come to us asking for help in distracting a child from pain, or to hold a hand during a scary procedure. The nurses believe strongly in my daily music therapy group and will find a way to bring their patients down to the playroom on time. If we know a patient loves the music therapy group, we will coordinate baths/respiratory therapy/medicines, etc. as much as we can to get the child there. On rare occasions I'll change the time for music therapy group for a patient, but that has its own consequences since so many other patients and nurses are counting on it to occur at 11:30 daily.

A simple way to create strong friendships with nursing staff is to have lunch with them. We eat in the nurses' report room/lounge. When I first started working on Pediatrics, the two Child Life specialists ate in their shoebox-sized office, and I ate with the nurses. I soon encouraged the Child Life staff to join us. It is very easy to harbor an us/them attitude in many facilities, but something as simple as eating together forces us to interact. And the nurses are really a wealth of information – I gain so much knowledge from them during lunch. It is also an informal way to network. We see the kids from different perspectives, and it's always valuable to gain someone else's insight.

I'll do anything

One reason I get along well with the nurses and Child Life staff is that I'll do anything for Pediatrics. If a nurse needs someone to hang out with a patient while a parent goes to the cafeteria, and it's during a time when no volunteer is around, I'm available. I'll hold cranky babies, I'll feed babies, I'll change diapers. As a music therapist, I can always sing to a baby, or dance her around the room in an effort to calm her. I've cleaned wagons before a state inspection. I sweep the playroom floor. I play games with kids. I watch kids play video games, but I am really too old to try to learn how to play them. Sometimes you just feel that a child wants you there. Your presence is requested.

One day I walked into the Child Life office and instead of their usual, "Good morning, Kathy," they asked, "Kathy, how tall are you?" Well, you know that's a bad sign. Apparently they'd arranged for the book and TV character "Arthur" the aardvark to come to the hospital, but somehow the actor inside the costume was unavailable. They needed someone of a certain height to volunteer to dress up and walk around the floor as the bespectacled aardvark. That's when I realized that I will truly do anything for Pediatrics.

It was actually a lot of fun going around in character. I knew which kids would love to give Arthur a hug, and which kids would rather I just keep moving, thank you very much. Unfortunately I couldn't wear my glasses under Arthur's huge head, so I was very visually challenged. This Arthur needed a guide dog. It also got very hot inside that costume and I prayed that Arthur wouldn't collapse in the playroom and require CPR (cardiopulmonary resuscitation) in front of the kids!

Among the written feedback I received after my presentation at a national American Music Therapy Association conference was the indignant remark: "Sometimes she doesn't even do music therapy with the children." That's right, folks. But I'll still wager that I have more hands-on therapy time with the kids than most music therapists in most facilities. In fact, I've met music therapists from state facilities who spend 20 hours/week in "activity therapy", and 20 hours/week on paperwork! That is outrageous to me, especially as a taxpayer. While I appreciate the value of justifying my existence at the hospital, I value my time with the children more. Therefore, since I created my job, I streamlined the paperwork demands to only that which is essential.

I also have the luxury of being on staff. If I were contracting music therapy services, I would feel compelled to do music therapy and only music therapy, since that was what the contract specified. Being a staff member, however, makes me free to do what is necessary at any given time. Our Pediatric floor functions like a giant beehive, with a lot of worker bees doing whatever job needs doing.

Before we had a playroom assistant, our Child Life department would take turns keeping the playroom open whenever our volunteers were on holidays. The playroom is vitally important to all of our younger kids and their families, and it does not diminish my role as a music therapist to do other activities with them if necessary. This includes playing house, drawing/painting at the tables (although the only thing I can draw is an elephant), chasing toddlers who are running away from their IV poles, and following a little one who is riding a toy car around the Pediatric floor. Believe me, it endears me to my coworkers if I'm willing to do these jobs, and it would not endear me to them if I insisted, "You know, that's not really in my job description."

There have been times when I've started a relationship with a child over keyboards, or singing together, or a little one who's loved the music therapy group, but over the years our friendship has evolved. I had a great patient with cystic fibrosis (CF) whom I knew for 11 years. She had always been in the music therapy group with her dad when she was little. Then I gave her keyboard lessons when she felt too old and sophisticated for the group. Then in her early teens she wanted the younger and cooler college volunteers to play board games with her. One day we had no volunteers. Since our kids with CF are routinely hospitalized for two to three weeks, that's a lot of time to get bored. So I went into her room and said, "Sorry, Terry, we're fresh out of volunteers. Are you desperate enough to play with me? We can play any game you choose." She chose Yahtzee (from Milton-Bradley) and from that moment on, over the next few years until her death, we had monster Yahtzee tournaments whenever she was hospitalized. Even though I am neither young nor hip, she'd gotten used to my sense of humor over the years, and these tournaments brought us even closer together. It wasn't the game, that was just a vehicle for us to get outrageously silly together. But laughing is wonderful therapy for anyone with a lung disease.

Sometimes I've worked with a patient on keyboards, and he's gotten tired of it and wanted to move on to something else. But if I got ready to leave, the child grabbed the keyboard desperately and said, "OK, I'll play it some more." Clearly he wanted to play something else with me. Should I tell this child, "Hey, I do music therapy or nothing," and walk out? If I feel that I'm on the verge of developing a therapeutic relationship with a child, I know I need to stay as long as it takes to clinch the deal. The kids I work with are oftentimes facing some very big challenges. Having a friend in the hospital is going to make that easier for everyone – the patient, family, and staff.

I have a patient who is now ten years old. Her parents are from Southeast Asia where they fled unspeakable atrocities and war. They spent years in a Thai refugee camp where they contracted HIV from acupuncture needles. Her mother lost two young sons due to starvation and disease in the jungle while fleeing the advancing North Vietnamese army. Reading the history in the chart and talking to her mother made me cry at night. I first met this patient when she was three years old. She was in for an extended stay and we became friends. Then she was in briefly when she was six. When she was nine, she was admitted again for three weeks, this time for full-blown AIDS. We'd always been friends, but now we recognized in each other a vast need for silliness. She would sit next to me during the music therapy group and watch me, waiting for me to make her laugh. Well, I do hate to disappoint my patients, and even if I just crossed my eyes at her, she'd double over laughing.

She was home for a month when she came back with a very bad pneumonia. She ended up on a ventilator in the Pediatric Intensive Care Unit (PICU). I went over every day to see her. Often I'll sing to my patients in the PICU, but for this girl I just talked to her (even though she was heavily sedated), held her hand, and listened to and hugged her mom, who wouldn't leave her bedside. Eventually the little girl got better. She was extubated (removed from the ventilator) and her medications decreased. But even though she could talk to us, she couldn't open her eyes. After a few days, the doctors pried her eyes open, and she was blind. The opportunistic infections that are the hallmark of AIDS (cyto-megalovirus and herpes) had attacked her retinas and left them detached.

My girl who had already been through so much in her short life, who had been to the brink of death and back, was now blind. So again, I cried. But we found a way to move on. And though it helped to have a special keyboard that let us record really stupid sounds and laugh over them, it helped even more for us to have a relationship already developed to get us both through this difficult time.

One afternoon I went to see her and had to wait for the nurses to hold her down for the dreaded eye drops. When they were done, she was still crying, but she heard my voice and we immediately went into our silliness mode. She literally stopped crying within seconds. She's such a humor addict – probably my easiest audience.

Her vision gradually got better in one eye, and I asked her,

"Can you see me?"

"Yes."

"Do I have three heads?"

She laughed. When this girl laughed, her whole body would get involved. She'd clasp her hands together, and fling her face away from me and toward her mother, who would laugh at her daughter's glee. Then she said,

"No, not three heads!"

"Oh, so only two heads, but six arms, right?"

Again, that physical laughter. When she faced me again, I milked it.

"So, two heads, six arms, and a tail, right?"
Don't be boring, and it's the relationship, stupid.

Support your local nurse!

Nursing is a brutal job. Nurses have to cause pain, and they have to hold down children for doctors to inflict pain. They have to deal with stressed parents, abusive parents, and screaming parents who may be in a custody battle over their hospitalized child. They also have to deal with doctors who come in all personality types: the new, the experienced, the forgetful, the obstinate, the ones who love and understand children, and the ones who don't. Nurses are also expected to protect children from unnecessary pain, even it if means contradicting a doctor. Doctors, of course, don't appreciate being contradicted, and though our head nurse will support our nurses in this endeavor, everyone knows the nurse could lose his or her job over this action.

Nurses have a tremendous amount of responsibility. They have to double-check every medication they give, because if a child gets the wrong amount, even if it's what the doctor ordered, it's the nurse's license that is on the line. Nurses also have to clean up copious amounts of bodily fluids that come out of every imaginable place. (Most of the time they measure it, too.) It is no wonder nurses flee their profession.

I believe that part of my job is to help our nursing staff whenever I can. How do I do that as a music therapist? Easy. I take all the "problem patients".

Hyperactive kids drive nurses crazy

Nurses are already busy, and having an especially busy child just adds to their craziness. Therefore, all hyperactive kids are automatically referred to me. You'd be surprised how many of these kids are hospitalized. Actually you shouldn't be – these are the ones who climb bookshelves, TVs, and filing cabinets before they learn how to walk. When they get older, they do Superman impersonations off the roof. Even without the naturally hyperactive segment of the population, the hospital has an amazing array of medicines that make even normally sedate kids bounce off the walls. There have been times when I've arrived at the playroom first thing in the morning to find kids ricocheting around, and volunteers and foster grandparents pulling their hair out with that dazed but desperate look in their eyes. On days like this I run a STAT (emergency) music therapy group. I throw drums onto the table, grab my guitar, clear my throat, and shout, "Hey! I've got some drums here. Anyone interested?" Usually there follows an enormous "whoosh" sound as the kids fly into chairs. They pick up drumsticks, someone closes the door, and we're off. We sing and drum until some of that energy is bled off. I can then return nearly civilized kids back to their nurses, the playroom volunteers decide not to quit that day after all, and the kids are no longer being yelled at. One thing continues to amaze me – hyperactive kids are almost always great drummers. They are also very appropriate in the music therapy group – well behaved and everything. I think it's because they've finally found a place that accepts them. They need to move and make noise, and I offer them the only forum in the hospital to do that. A lot of folks don't see drums as a socializing/civilizing tool. Music therapists do.

Special populations have special needs

Many of these kids can be frequent flyers to the hospital. Children with cerebral palsy come in for orthopedic problems and aspiration pneumonia. Patients with spina bifida (or myelomeningocele, my favorite word) are hospitalized for shunt revisions for their hydrocephalus (water on the brain), or urinary tract infections that require IV antibiotics. Kids with Down syndrome not only have heart problems, they are, unfortunately, more likely to develop leukemia than the normal population. Special kids seem more susceptible to the big bad germs in the world at large – pneumonia, flu, and diarrhea. They get knocked down more easily, and it takes a longer time for them to build back up again. Surgery really can throw them for a loop. Some of these kids just seem more fragile all the way around. If it's important for normal kids to have supportive relationships when they're hospitalized, it's even more critical for the special population. Some of these kids live in group homes, and it's difficult for their caretakers to be at their bedside. Even if they have loving families, the folks of these children may face more stress than other parents. If this is the first time the child has been in this hospital, there's a lot of educating the staff. What is baseline for this child? Is he verbal? Can she walk/crawl/roll/move both sides of her body?

There may also be subtle and not-so-subtle prejudices against the special population. Nurses might think it's an extra chore to put a child with cerebral palsy into his wheelchair so that he can attend the music therapy group. It helps to give the nurse advanced warning. An hour before group, I'll find the nurse and say, "You know, Bobby is so great in the music therapy group. He just lights up the room with that beautiful smile. Do you think we could get him down to the playroom at 11:30?" If you give people enough warning, it's more difficult for them to think of an excuse why they can't do it. If the nurse sees how Bobby comes alive when he gets to the playroom, chances are good that she will become more bonded to him. Then she'll make sure Bobby gets to the playroom in time for music in the future.

Parents of these kids also have to contend with hospital staff who may feel their child's life is not as important as others. One of my favorite kids ended up on a ventilator in the PICU after surgery for a gastric-tube (feeding tube) revision. He developed respiratory complications and was fighting for his life. His mother faced some horrible decisions: "Should I make him a DNR status (Do Not Resuscitate)? Is this his time to die? Am I putting him through extra misery just for me?" The intensive care staff had never met this boy before. They didn't know that this child had given his mother the courage to leave an abusive husband, or that his brother and two sisters depended upon him. This child, who couldn't walk or talk, somehow stabilized an otherwise chaotic household environment. The PICU nurses saw him as a seven-year-old boy, severely afflicted with cerebral palsy, and now close to death. To some of them, there was no question that he should be made a DNR status. Unfortunately, the mother overheard such a conversation, grew angry and resentful, and lost confidence in these nurses.

This boy eventually recovered and returned to his treasured position in his family. Somehow, as severe as his cerebral palsy is, he is still one of the silliest and happiest kids I've ever met. He has a smile that can very nearly crumble brick.

Priority patients

Other children who are a priority for music therapy include kids at both extremes of the energy continuum (hyperactive and comatose), kids stuck in isolation, kids with no family around, terrified kids, and kids in traction. Children are also stuck in their beds when they come in for days of EEG (electro-encephalograph) monitoring. These are usually patients who have seizures that the medical staff wants to document. The EEG technician will tape several electrical leads to the child's head and run them to the EEG machine. The child will also be monitored by videotape, so when you work with such a child, you'll be on camera, too! Now most of the time, this strategy works as well as when your car has a constant funny noise that stops as soon as you take it to the mechanic, or when your child has a fever that goes away the moment you step into the pediatrician's office. That's right. Children rarely have seizures when they're being monitored on the EEG machine!

One day our Pediatric floor was visited by two of my favorite characters: Elmo and Cookie Monster from *Sesame Street*. They couldn't talk, but they were really nuts. After playing with the kids in the playroom, I took them to visit a boy I knew who was stuck in 48-hour EEG monitoring. Elmo leapt onto the bed with the child as I explained the concept of the video camera to Cookie Monster. He immediately thrust his crazy oogely eyes in front of the camera and started shaking them around. His blue furry body completely filled the video screen, and I remember thinking, I'd give good money to watch the neurologists as they review this tape.

Hierarchy

There are times when our census (pediatric population in the hospital) is low, and staff and volunteers pile up on the same kids – whatever kids happen to be awake! This doesn't happen very often, but it can be a problem. There is a hierarchy to be observed in a hospital. For instance, it's more important for the medical and nursing staff to see a child than for me. So if I'm working with a child and the doctor comes in, I'll ask if I should come back later. Sometimes the doctor needs to physically examine the child, and I'll leave for privacy. Many times the doctor will say, "I'll only be a few minutes," so I'll wait outside the door. If a nurse or respiratory therapist is working with a child, I'll poke my head into the room and ask, "How long are you going to be busy with Roberto?" When a child is being followed by a lot of therapies (physical, occupational, speech), Child Life will make up a chart and we all work together to schedule ourselves in.

The important thing is to be polite and respectful of the other services. There is also a lot of give and take. If the art therapist gives up her time with a child due to my halftime schedule, I'll be sure to accommodate her the next time she needs it. Sometimes the kids will make the call for you. If two staff members show up at the same time in a patient's room, an assertive child will settle the matter by pointing – "You can stay, and you can come back later." Kids can be devastatingly honest. Life on Pediatrics is humbling! Unless, of course, they pick you!

Families are also more important than me, particularly a family that is not usually at the bedside. This is a delicate balance. I'm not going to get in the way between a child and his family because that is very powerful therapy in its own right. However, if this is a family that is in frequently, I'm not seen as an interruption but as a diversion, an opportunity to play together as a family. I'll also take care of the patient and siblings while the parents take a break. It's important for the family to know that if they can't be at the bedside, someone is laughing and playing with their child. There's an African proverb: "It takes a village to raise a child." In this circumstance, it takes a village to help a child and family cope with hospitalization.

Be kind to housekeepers

I am friends with all of our housekeepers. I bring them cookies at Christmas, and persimmons and pomegranates from my trees in the fall. Our housekeepers work hard and have a tough job, with menial pay. If you are kind to the housekeepers, they will be kind to you, and you will have the help you need when a child throws up in the playroom.

Our housekeepers get very close to the families of frequently hospitalized kids, as do the cafeteria workers who deliver their meals and snacks each day, and the patient escort staff who takes them to radiology, etc. These staff members may need support when a child they know goes to the PICU or is dying. I make sure these staff members are aware of any transfers to the PICU and offer to go with them to visit a child. Sometimes these folks are so depressed over the loss of a patient that they have to transfer off the Pediatric floor for a while. But this is the type of employee we want to keep on Pediatrics, so all of us try to support the ancillary staff members to keep them around.

These extra employees are also handy to use as vocal back-ups. Years ago, it just so happened that I'd be working with a little girl in the PICU at the same time the chaplain (who I later found out was an undercover nun!) would visit and the housekeeper cleaned her room. Daily we met and performed the greatest "Supreme" impersonations you could ever hope to see. We were dynamite! The girl loved us and we loved us.

Housekeepers (and chaplains) are our friends and sometimes function well as the "Pips." (Remember Gladys Knight and the Pips?) So, if you're working with a patient who has no roommate, and the extra bed looks neat and clean, it is. Please do not mess it up by putting your extra equipment and stuff on the nice, clean bed. A roommate may show up at any moment and will want a pristine bed. Also do not put your equipment on top of the laundry containers or trash receptacles. (These are requirements of the Joint Commission on the Accreditation of Health Organizations.)

MT assessment – what do you really need to know?

Music therapists tend to like assessments that are of the fill-in-the-blanks variety. They want to get all the information they need and cover all the bases. Unfortunately in the environment of an acute medical setting, things move very quickly. When I first stepped onto the Pediatric floor, the level of stress was so palpable that I feared it might overwhelm me. Now of course, I'm immersed in the flow. I've developed the classic run/walk characteristic of Pediatrics staff. Visitors and interns comment on how fast we all walk as they run to keep up with us. We don't even notice it anymore. We run between patients so that we can spend more time when we're with them.

Teaching hospitals are wonderful in that there is tremendous expertise from many different specialties under one roof. The downside is that it drives patients and parents crazy when they have to answer the same questions over and over again as each new specialty service comes on board for a referral. Then of course, within each specialty there is the medical student, the resident, and the attending physician, each with their own repeating set of questions.

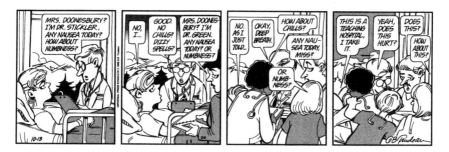

Doonesbury copyright © 1995 G.B. Trudeau. Reprinted with permission of Universal Press Syndicate. All rights reserved.

We don't need to add to this problem. So, referral and data collection forms must be quick and painless. Of course, in any new program you want documentation to justify someone paying for your services. However, I've looked at some music therapy referral forms and thought, "My nurses simply don't have time to fill that out". In the acute medical setting these days, patients are sicker, hospitals are downsizing, and nurses have ever-increasing responsibilities. I want to make their job easier, not give them more to do.

Since I work under the Child Life department, I am covered by the blanket order that allows me to see every child on Pediatrics. Every morning, the Child Life folks leave me a printout of the census for the general pediatric floor and the PICU. It lists the information I need such as:

- name
- diagnosis
- primary medical service (Neuro, Rehab, Renal, Pulmonary, etc.)
- admitting doctor
- number of days the child has been hospitalized
- isolation codes (more on this later).

The Child Life specialists work fulltime and arrive early to go to surgery with kids. They get additional information from the Rand (aka, cardex) – this is a flip-up system containing a large card on each patient. The Rand contains vital information that is updated daily. My coworkers will amend my census to include:

- nicknames
- primary language spoken by child and parents
- ambulatory status (wheelchair, cardiac chair, wagon, etc.)
- activity level (playroom, bedrest, out of bed 3x/day, etc.)
- unique features of the child (developmentally delayed, blind, nonverbal, etc.)
- expected procedures during the day (operating room – OR, CT, magnetic resonance imaging – MRI)
- allergies (latex, milk, etc.)
- dietary restrictions (NPO – *nil per os* – nothing by mouth).

They will also mention kids who may need special attention because:

- no family at bedside
- hyperactive – driving nurses crazy
- combative – hit nurse last night
- in traction – maybe we can move bed to playroom
- birthday/last day of chemo/discharge from rehab – needs a party
- anxious – needs guided imagery/relaxation training
- new diagnosis, or awaiting test results (cancer suspected).

So, I can get a lot of information without asking the family a single question. Then it's easy for a nurse to stop me in the hallway and say, "If you have time, could you check in with Billy in room 65? He's had a miserable morning with lots of procedures and could really use some cheering up."

There are situations when you simply don't have time to read the chart or get much information from the nurse. Once a nurse asked me to go see a scared 12-year-old boy who'd just been transferred to the PICU for a bronchoscopy (where a tube is inserted down the esophagus). The nurse barely knew the boy. He'd gotten a piece of meat stuck in his throat

– luckily he was able to breathe around it, but was unable to dislodge it himself. Now he was going to the PICU for the procedure under sedation. No Child Life specialists were around, and the nurse was concerned that the boy's anxiety would escalate. I didn't have time to even grab a tape recorder for guided imagery. Luckily he and his mom were easily distracted by humor and we told jokes and silly stories while waiting for the doctors to get their equipment organized. It sure beat letting this boy go crazy with fear sitting in an intensive care unit wondering what was going to happen.

Oftentimes I think that over the course of my career on Pediatrics, my assessment has boiled down to two questions:

1. Who is screaming now?
2. Can I help?

Data collection – less is more

Again, paperwork must be quick and painless. You also need to get the big picture. During my internship at a small hospital, my supervisor told me to enter a patient's room with all of my senses alert and ready to take in everything that's going on around me. That includes the behavior not only of the child, but also of the family members and staff in the room. My personal feeling is that if you are totally focused on counting specific behaviors, you run the risk of not seeing the forest for the trees. Stay alert to what's going on in the group or the individual child in front of you. Be here now! Being fully available to your patient will promote a more positive interaction. If necessary, make short notes after you leave a patient.

Patient/parent satisfaction surveys are great, but keep in mind that a parent is very anxious to get home. I've known parents of frequently hospitalized kids who will leave at 3:00 am and drive over mountain passes in the snow to get home after discharge! The parents of kids coming in for routine chemo actually count the hours until they can go home. They become impatient if the chemo isn't started as soon as they arrive because everything is delayed from that point on. So if you need a survey filled out by parents, make sure you get it to them early.

Regarding statistics, our Child Life department used to keep lots of them. We kept track of how many children we saw each day, what activities we did with each one, how much time we spent on each interaction, who referred each child to us, etc. After several years of recording this data, piling up impressive numbers, and our supervisor dutifully filing reports full of them, we finally asked – who is reading these reports? Well, it turned out nobody was. We talked with our administrator, who gave us permission to stop keeping the data. That was actually a little scary – doing our jobs without obsessing about numbers. It was like working without a net. We were so programmed into keeping statistics because we thought it showed how important our work was. It didn't – especially if no one bothered to read the reports. Now we have more time to spend with the children, instead of wasting time keeping data. Keep in mind that ours is a well-established program and we did put in years of keeping data. We may also have a more enlightened administrator who believes strongly in our Child Life department – we don't have to convince her. (I warned you in the beginning that I may not do things the way you were taught in school. Think about it, though – if the foundation for your program is built upon paperwork, just how strong is that foundation?)

Charting

One of my interns came with a tendency to write chart notes like: "Bobby shook the maraca 3x, and looked at me 4x. He seemed happy as evidenced by smiling 2x." I gently explained to her that in many facilities that would be absolutely appropriate, but here, "Ain't nobody gonna read that, honey." It'll put them to sleep before they get past the first maraca shake. My note on the same event may read: "Bobby seemed rather quiet in the playroom until we started MT group where he demonstrated considerable prowess on conga drum and maracas. He was very interactive with staff and other kids. Will continue to offer MT group as a means of venting emotions/energy." One important aspect to charting is that the medical staff will see that Bobby behaves very differently in the music therapy group than when they examine him. For them, Bobby is a terrified, silent child – for me, Bobby is a maniac drummer.

I've seen sample music therapy notes that filled up half a page in the chart. If I write a note that long it means something is very wrong, i.e., I'm worried about a two-year-old being discharged home with an inattentive family and IV antibiotics and back up that concern by describing their interactions that I've witnessed in the playroom and patient's room. If I have these types of concerns, not only do I chart them, I also notify the social worker and patient's nurse directly.

Chart notes need to be short, sweet, and to the point, preferably without jargon that may be an attempt to impress the reader with our intelligence. Sometimes, as music therapists, we think we know what the medical community wants: numbers and strictly objective observations. However, I've been working in a teaching hospital for a long time and I'm finding that the medical community doesn't expect us to cram something as creative as music therapy into a test tube. They respect it because although it is completely different from their approach, it's making their patients and families happy. It's making kids laugh while they're in a hospital undergoing painful procedures and taking yucky medicines. And in the process, it's making everyone's lives easier – nurses, doctors, patients and parents. In this setting, that is just a little shy of a miracle.

Rounds

Lots of rounds take place in a hospital. This is where the doctors, residents, medical students, nurses, etc. meet to discuss each patient on their service. Each service has its own rounds – Rehabilitation, Neurology, Pediatrics, Pulmonary, etc. It's great if you can find an inter-disciplinary group that will meet at least weekly to fill you in on patients on the Pediatric floor and PICU. We discovered Discharge Planning Rounds, which used to meet twice weekly, but due to budget cuts and lay-offs has been reduced to once a week. This group is comprised of the discharge planner (a nurse), the charge nurse (who decides which child goes into which room and maintains nurse/patient staffing ratios), physical therapy, occupational therapy, Child Life, art therapy, music therapy, and a social worker. It is fundamentally a forum to discuss discharge needs, but since they go over every patient on the floor, we pick up a lot of information on current kids. It is very insightful to gain perspectives from the other disciplines – it leads to a more unified approach. If we have a child who is a bit of a behavior challenge, or a parent with a borderline personality disorder, it pays to have everyone approaching the problem from a similar angle.

Again, the nurses have a lot of knowledge about diseases and medicines that can be very valuable to us. The doctors' rounds, however, will be geared to the residents and medical students, and will really be over the head of anyone who missed more than two days of medical school. So find a group that will let you in and start learning.

Changing the environment

One of the more wonderful aspects of having music therapy at a hospital is hearing live music in the hallways. We have children singing and drumming in the daily group; guitar music and lullabies coming from the baby rooms; flute sounds whenever I had interns (somehow both of my interns played flute); and kids practicing keyboard in their rooms. These sounds tend to counteract the sterility and foreign feeling of the hospital environment, and promote a further level of normalcy. Plus, everyone in the hallway starts smiling.

Once we had a ten-year-old boy with leukemia. He'd recently seen a group of actors who'd come to his school from the cast of *The Phantom of the Opera* (Webber 1993). It had made a huge impression on him, and he was full of the songs and drama from the show. He had already learned some tunes on the keyboard with me, so I brought out my biggest keyboard and taught him how to play the beginning of Bach's Toccata in D minor – the spooky music from the original movie. He learned it quickly and practiced often. Then the art therapist helped him make a phantom facemask out of plaster casting material. The effect was complete. People walking down the hallway would hear the haunting pipe organ music and then, if they were brave enough to poke their heads into the room, they'd see a boy sitting on the bed wearing his phantom mask. It was perfect.

5. Getting Specific in the Acute Medical Setting

Common diseases in pediatrics

Sickle cell anemia

Sickle cell anemia is a hereditary disease that affects predominantly people of African-Caribbean descent. Normal red blood cells are round and flexible. They slip through small capillaries with ease and supply all the parts of the body with oxygen. However, when red blood cells sickle, a percentage of these normally round cells collapse in on themselves, forming a crescent moon shape. This shape is not conducive to flow and instead forms "log-jams" in small capillaries. It is also not effective at transporting oxygen throughout the body. Blood cells can sickle and block the circulatory system anywhere, and can cause extremely swollen limbs. Sickling cells in the brain can cause CVA (cerebrovascular accident, or stroke). In the lungs, these cells can cause "acute chest syndrome", where virtually no air is moving in the lungs. These patients frequently end up on a ventilator in the PICU.

When patients with sickle cell anemia are admitted to the hospital it is almost always due to "pain crisis." These kids are in tremendous pain, which can migrate throughout their bodies. Often narcotics are employed to combat the pain, but it can be a balancing act to find the dose that will cover the pain without causing the patient to slip into respiratory failure. Treatment also includes blood transfusions to dilute the sickle cells. Frequently our kids will have a "designated donor" at the blood bank – a person in the community who is a good match and has agreed to come in frequently to supply our patient when blood is needed. Sickle cell anemia is a very frightening and depressing disease for our children. It can cripple our kids and even cause death. Stem cell transplant is becoming an option for some patients with sickle cell anemia.

Cystic fibrosis

This is also a hereditary disease, this time predominantly affecting the white community. It mainly damages lungs, but can also play a substantial gastro-intestinal role. In cystic fibrosis (CF), the mucous is much thicker than normal and is difficult to clear from the lungs. The gastro-intestinal tract isn't as efficient at digesting food, and the kids have to take supplemental enzymes. Often a gastric tube is surgically placed so the patients can get supplemental feeds directly to their stomachs while they sleep because they just can't get enough calories orally.

CF is a demanding disease that requires daily respiratory therapy treatments be done at home. Our kids with CF are routinely hospitalized for a three-week "tune-up" where they are given intravenous antibiotics and round-the-clock respiratory therapy treatments. Any little cold can also slam these kids back in the hospital. The CF cough is a true bone-rattler, and it can give you pause to hear it. These kids frequently contract various organisms that are resistant to certain antibiotics, like pseudomonas and MRSA (methicillin resistant staphylococcus aureus). Unfortunately, this can lead to them being stuck in isolation for the duration of their hospital stay. This isn't so bad for the teenagers, but it's horrible for younger kids who are in love with the playroom. CF is a terminal disease. Although kids are living longer now than they were 20 years ago, there still is no cure. And these kids know that. Lung transplants are becoming more of an option these days, but the body still creates the sticky mucous that will eventually destroy the new lungs as well.

Cancers in children

Unfortunately, cancer is not just an old person's disease – it also attacks and kills children. Whereas an adult may grow a tumor over a 10–20 year time period before it becomes a problem, children are programmed for growth. Tumors in children grow so quickly that by the time they're even noticeable, they've often metastasized (sent out malignant cells into the bloodstream that are now growing in another part of the body). This makes them very difficult to treat. Tumors are frequently misdiagnosed in children because the average pediatrician and family practitioner are not looking for them. This also increases the time where the tumor is growing unchecked.

Cancerous tumors can grow anywhere – in the brain, bones, muscles, organs. Brain tumors are actually one of the most common cancers in children. Kids will present with horrible headaches, inconsolable crying, vomiting, dizziness, or an off-balance gait. Treatment for brain tumors can be challenging. There is a blood-brain barrier that flows below the brain, protecting it from many outside agents that may affect the rest of the body. Some chemotherapy won't cross the blood-brain barrier, leaving surgery and radiation as the modalities of choice. However, in small children (under five years old) both of these interventions can cause tremendous damage in a developing brain. Doctors and parents may be faced with a horrendous dilemma – a child who will die without treatment, or a child who may be severely brain damaged as a result of treatment. Children who have surgery for excision (removal) of brain tumors will sometimes need inpatient rehabilitation afterward to help them cope with the deficits incurred as a result of the surgery.

Bone tumors present with limb pain, broken bones (because the tumor actually causes a pathological fracture), and kids who suddenly cannot walk. The tumors are frequently shrunk with chemotherapy as much as possible and then amputated. An alternative to amputation that is sometimes possible is called "limb salvage". In this surgery, the affected bone is removed and a titanium rod is put in its place. This is certainly more cosmetic, but it has inherent problems in children who may still be growing. Future surgeries will be required to accommodate growth to match the opposite limb. The salvaged limb will also be more fragile than before. Amputation has its own problems, with body image issues and problems with phantom limb pain.[1] Another side effect of chemotherapy, besides suppressing the immune system, is slowing the healing process. So it can take a while for the amputated stump to heal. One positive

---

1   Phantom limb pain is a phenomenon in which the patient still feels pain in
     the limb that was amputated. It can be quite severe over the course of the year
     following amputation.

aspect to amputation is that we are living in an age of constantly improving prosthetic devices. Kids have returned to the hospital for visits and to show off their new and improved artificial legs. We have a photograph of one of our patients, a 12-year-old girl who underwent a lower leg amputation, in her blue sequined costume and tap shoes after her dance recital. Her new leg even has a synthetic covering that looks and almost feels like skin. She is one of our favorite success stories.

Leukemia is the most common cancer in children. Luckily the form referred to as "childhood leukemia" (acute lymphocytic leukemia, or ALL) has an 80 per cent cure rate. That's *cure*, not just remission. Of course, those patients are followed in the outpatient clinic, where cancer is treated like a chronic disease, and after their years of treatment are over, they go on with their normal lives. Those are not the patients I see in the hospital. The ones I work with are the unlucky ones in that 20 per cent category – the kids who relapse and don't respond well to the treatment. I also see the kids who are diagnosed with other types of leukemia that have much lower cure rates.

Leukemia is a blood cancer that can present in all kinds of ways – an ear infection that will not heal, a nosebleed that won't stop, a menstrual period that won't end, a respiratory infection that won't go away, a white pallor to the skin. The bone marrow, which is the body's blood factory, stops producing mature blood cells. So the white blood cells that usually fight off infection are no longer working effectively. Platelets are unable to clot to stop bleeding. The red blood cells that are produced are inefficient at transporting oxygen throughout the body, no longer giving cheeks a rosy glow. Platelets and red blood cells can be transfused into patients, but the white blood cells are too fragile to transfuse. Chemotherapy also reduces the supply of white blood cells, leaving patients with neutropenia (low counts of the right kind of blood cells) and heightened susceptibility to whatever germ is passing by.

Children diagnosed with cancer of any type are subjected to many strenuous and invasive procedures. They are poked for blood multiple times, forced to submit to many different types of scans (CT, MRI, bone scans, brain scans), and have to undergo lumbar punctures (spinal taps) and bone marrow aspirations just for the initial diagnosis of cancer. In a bone marrow aspiration the child is sedated and the doctor uses a large gauge needle to penetrate the pelvic bone and withdraw bone marrow.

Sometimes the bone marrow is so packed with immature blood cells that it can be difficult to even pull back on the syringe to withdraw the fluid. In this case, a bone marrow biopsy is required, where a bigger piece of the bone marrow is removed for examination under the microscope.

Chemotherapy, radiation, and surgery are the modalities used to treat cancer. There are several different chemotherapeutic agents that are used alone and in conjunction with each other and radiation to combat these mutant cells. Cancer cells are fast growing and chemotherapy attacks fast growing cells. Unfortunately hair cells and cells that line the gastro-intestinal tract (mouth to anus) are also fast growing and therefore killed off as a side effect. Children lose their hair to a greater or lesser degree. Some are absolutely bald, without eyebrows or even eyelashes. Others, with exceptionally thick hair, may lose some or even just a little. Vomiting used to be a tremendous problem with chemotherapy, but there have been some amazing drug advances that have solved that problem for most patients. A big problem for children is mouth sores. Kids suffer from lesions that can populate the mouth and run all the way down the esophagus to the stomach. This is horribly painful and is treated with morphine or other narcotics, as well as mouth care rinses.

It is amazing that children facing such tremendous challenges can still want to play. But they do. Children newly diagnosed with cancer will go down to the operating room in the early morning, get a broviac catheter placed (which will make everybody's life easier because it greatly reduces the number of required pokes), and be ready to cruise the playroom in the afternoon. Sometimes they've been in my music therapy group at 11:30! Kids recover more quickly than adults, and are usually in a hurry to get back to the important basics of being a kid – play.

Bone marrow transplant/stem cell transplant

Bone marrow transplant/stem cell transplant (BMT/SCT) is a treatment for certain kinds of cancers and is also becoming an option for some patients with sickle cell anemia. Bone marrow is harvested from the patient, or from a donor whose blood is a close match. Stem cells are harvested from the patient in a process called "pheresis" using a machine that looks a lot like a kidney dialysis machine. Stem cells can also be harvested from an umbilical cord if the patient's mom is pregnant and will be delivering soon. If a patient's own bone marrow is to be used for the transplant, the marrow is purged with radiation and chemotherapy to kill off any cancerous cells before being returned to the patient. Stem cells are preferable because the harvesting technique is easier for the donor. Although pheresis requires hours of lying in bed to get a sufficient amount of viable blood cells, the alternative is undergoing dozens of bone marrow aspirations with that large bore needle into the pelvis in the operating room. There is a fair amount of pain in the recovery. Sometimes the oncologist will prefer one method over the other for medical reasons.

In BMT/SCT, the patient undergoes total body irradiation and increased doses of chemotherapy in an effort to kill off any cancerous cells in the body. It is a full body assault. After several days of radiation and chemotherapy, the bone marrow is dripped into the patient by transfusion. Then everyone waits for the new bone marrow to engraft into the patient and start producing healthy blood cells. Since the patient is so beaten down with radiation and chemotherapy, complications are almost to be expected. These can range from mild to fatal and include infection, organ failure, and graft versus host disease (GVHD). GVHD can affect any organ system. A little of it is a good thing – it means the graft is working – but a lot can kill a patient.

Patients who are undergoing BMT/SCT are the most immune compromised people on the planet. You would *never* visit them if you have even a sore throat or runny nose because that could actually kill them. Even if you think you're just suffering from allergies, don't go in. Most facilities require that only brand new, wrapped-in-plastic toys go into a BMT/SCT room. I have a stash of small, new keyboards and drums for that purpose. These patients are frequently very ill, but I did have a patient who felt great during her transplant. Her biggest problem was cabin fever, which can be very intense. They are truly stuck in their rooms for a couple of months.

Isolation

Isolation codes: it is essential to know the codes for your facility. At our hospital, kids on contact isolation are not allowed in our playroom. Contact implies that whatever they touch can be contagious. They are frequently feeling OK and will need lots of attention in their rooms. Take in drums or keyboards that are easy to rub down with a germicide after your sessions.

Respiratory isolation (from germs that are airborne) requires double door isolation rooms. This means that you go through one door into the anteroom, wait for that door to close all the way behind you, then go through the next door into the patient's room. Make sure you never have the two doors open at the same time because that is how nasty germs get into the hallway and travel to another patient.

Different bugs require different isolation precautions. Tuberculosis requires a special mask plus gown and gloves; chicken pox requires that you gown and glove with a less intense mask. Singing under these conditions can really make you want to faint, but resist this temptation because the child is probably very bored and desperate for some interaction. Isolation equipment (gowns, gloves, etc.) are taken off in the anteroom (if double door isolation) or in the patient's room (single door) and disposed of in the proper receptacle (probably the big red container that's labeled "Biohazardous material").

Isolation codes vary among institutions so be sure to follow the rules carefully. When in doubt, find a nurse and ask. These isolation codes keep germs from spreading through the hospital. Reverse isolation is for patients who are at risk for germs spreading to them – think BMT/SCT. Always remember to clean your instruments before going on to another patient.

By the way, people who wash their hands two hundred times a day are considered to be obsessive/compulsive unless they work in a hospital – then it's considered a good technique.

Latex allergies

One *very* important thing to note is if a child is allergic to latex. We do not even allow latex balloons on our floor. So many of our patients with spina bifida[2] have developed latex allergies that it's probably safest to just

2   Spina bifida is a birth defect in which the base of the neural tube is incompletely covered to a greater or lesser degree. It is frequently accompanied by hydrocephalus, requiring a shunt that reroutes fluid from the brain to the abdominal cavity where the body can eliminate it. Sometimes the defect causes incontinence, requiring the use of a catheter to empty the bladder.

assume all of that population is either allergic now or soon will be. Kids who are exposed to latex frequently (e.g. in urinary catheterization) can develop allergic reactions that range from mild to full blown anaphylactic shock[3]. Our nurses are also developing the allergy so our hospital has switched to vinyl gloves. All of our patients with spina bifida (aka, myelomeningocele) are now routinely tested for this allergy, so it is known they're allergic before they're even showing any symptoms. Latex is a soft rubber substance that can be found on the buttons (not the keys) of your portable keyboards, and on soft-headed drum mallets. For these kids, I either push the keyboard buttons myself, or give them a wooden drumstick to push with.

Child abuse

A word needs to be said about child abuse. Sometimes children are so badly abused, physically or sexually, that they need to be hospitalized. This stirs up a lot of emotions in the pediatric staff. It's hard enough to see kids suffering from the effects of accidents and disease – situations that are frequently unavoidable. But child abuse is optional – it does not have to happen. Most of the time, staff does not know who was the perpetrator of the crime against the child – it could be the mother, the father, mom's boyfriend or, indeed, the babysitter. Sometimes the child is old enough to tell the authorities what happened. The important thing is to focus on the child. It pushes all of our staff to the limits of our professionalism to be polite to the parents of obviously abused children, but it is not our place to judge them. Just focus on the child.

---

3   Anaphylactic shock is a catastrophic allergic reaction that can kill a person in five minutes unless epinephrine is administered. It is the response that kills people who are allergic to bee stings.

6. Tools of
the Trade

Piano lessons

I am fundamentally a piano player. I taught piano privately for ten years, both in classes and individually. I give a lot of lessons at the hospital. Physical therapy's criterion for discharge from the hospital has long been, can this child ambulate? My criterion for discharge is, can this child play *Happy Birthday* (Hill and Hill 1934)? I want them to be a hit at parties.

I find that teaching short, easy tunes by rote to kids is a lot of fun, increases their self-esteem (we love to perform for other staff), and gives the chronically ill kids a skill that they can continue to work on during future visits to the hospital. I teach a lot of duets so we can be silly together.

Keyboards are great because they're portable, they make a lot of interesting sounds, they're fairly cheap so when a kid pulls a key off I don't lose my mind, and they're easily cleaned. They also have a volume control, although every child (I don't care how delayed they may be) seems to figure out how to put the volume up to full blast just after they learn how to roll over. (It must be one of those developmental milestones.) So I find keyboards easier to use than say, trumpets, bassoons or bagpipes.

When teaching kids simple tunes, I am constantly aware that it needs to be a successful endeavor. I'm not going to let them feel like a failure because they just can't get *Twinkle Twinkle Little Star*. This can be difficult because I can't tell just by looking at a child if she will get it easily or really have a hard time. Kids have very different learning styles, and then we add in an assortment of interesting medicines that can slow them down or speed them up. Albuterol is a common medicine for kids with lung and airway problems. It is also notorious for raising energy levels so that kids are bouncing off the walls. You can always tell who's on Albuterol in the playroom! Teaching a tune to a kid on Albuterol is like throwing a piece of paper up into a tornado. It blows around violently with tremendous energy, and then somehow the kid absorbs the tune while you sit there feeling exhausted with the effort.

Likewise, kids who are on morphine or other narcotics for pain control can be challenging to try to teach. Sometimes they're so used to the medicine that they appear to be fairly normal. It's only when you see them trying to process new information that you notice something's taking a little longer than usual to crank through. If I suggest we try something else, they'll frequently say, "No, I know I can get this!" I'll say, "I know you can, but that morphine's in the way."

If I sense that learning a tune is just too difficult, I gently encourage the child to push some buttons and we simply enjoy exploring the sounds on the keyboard.

One interesting phenomenon that comes up repeatedly in my work is the necessity to play my instruments backwards, or even upside down (the instruments, not me). This was never presented in school that I can recall. But oftentimes I'll be teaching a child some little tune and it'll just be easier for me to play it upside down, without repositioning the keyboard. This happens with guitar as well. The patient and I are frequently facing each other, rather than sitting side by side. (Sometimes there is just not enough room to sit next to each other.) My former intern told me she has experienced the same phenomenon. She and a child shared her flute in the PICU. The music therapist blew into the mouthpiece from the opposite side while the child fingered the keys. So this is not unique to me, and I believe music therapy professors do their students a disservice by not requiring them to practice their instruments upside down and backwards. Don't let this happen to you! Be prepared.

Songwriting

Creating your own song is rewarding and therapeutic. It's a positive way to vent emotions. Somehow putting feelings into a song is easier than talking about those same feelings. It's also one of the few products we get in music therapy – something we can give to the family of a child with a horrible diagnosis.

Songwriting is a skill that I admire a great deal – this is because it's quite challenging for me. I do not consider myself among the great songwriters in music therapy. However, I recently found a wonderful nine-year-old girl who just loved my songs. She made me sing them with her whenever we got together. So I'm including some here in her honor, and to get my songs published!

Writing songs with children can range from the short and simple mad-libs to elaborate spill-your-guts original masterpieces. A very simple mad-lib that everyone knows, and therefore easy to implement, is *Yankee Doodle* (traditional).

Yankee Doodle went to (your favorite place)
Riding on a (anything – car, elephant, magic carpet, etc.)
Stuck a feather in his (article of clothing)
And called it (your favorite food).

The next rung up on the challenging songwriting ladder is using a familiar song with your own lyrics. This song came to me as I was playing ball in the house with my dog. (Isn't this the house you wish you grew up in?) I started writing it on the bus going into work, and finished it with a very creative patient. I used the melody of *My Favorite Things* (Rodgers and Hammerstein 1959).

Golden Retrievers on hard wooden floors,
Slipping and sliding they bash into doors,
Soft golden hair and fur float on the breeze,
Clinging to clothes and then making me sneeze.

Dogs who drink water and then drool and slobber;
Drips on the toes of my son and my daughter.
Chasing his tail and scratching at fleas,
Sniffing at hydrants and lampposts and trees.

When the dog snores, when the dog sheds,
When he rolls in slime,

> *I simply remember he could be a cat,*
> *And then I just feel so fine!*

Obviously the therapeutic value of this song is to create an opportunity to laugh and to vent my emotions of not being overly fond of cats.

This next song was written in a small group with a couple of ten-year-olds. Writing in a group situation, with a time limit because lunch was coming in ten minutes, was very intimidating for a songwriter like me. There was a lot of background noise and kid energy going on while I was trying to figure out a melody and chords for the words they'd just come up with. But these two kids both had pet iguanas, which are not exactly common as pets, and I just couldn't pass up an opportunity like that. One iguana was named "Bob" and he was vicious. The other iguana was named "Demon" and he was, of course, sweet. This tune is *Rock Around the Clock* (Myers and Freedman 1953).

> *Bob, Bob, Bob, Bob, Bob Iguana (repeat two more times)*
> *Oh, I've got an iguana and his name is Bob!*
> *Oh, Bob he snarls, and he growls,*
> *He walks like a little tiny dinosaur,*
> *Sometimes he bites, when he wears blue tights,*
> *But mostly he eats everything in sight,*
> *He's my prehistoric lizard and I love him with all my might.*

One benefit of writing a song with a child is the connection you build from working and creating together. Every time you see that child in the future she will demand that you sing the song together, and will probably request to write even more songs with you. Keeping a notebook of patients' songs is handy.

Song choosing

Children will sometimes choose songs that provide a means of communicating feelings. A five-year-old buddy of mine was waiting at the bus stop for me with his dad one morning. This little guy was excited about his plan to make a tape of his favorite songs, and he wanted me to help him. I ran up to the Pediatric floor, grabbed a tape recorder and cassette and ran back outside. We shooed his father away (to create the surprise!) and this little guy sang into the microphone in his husky voice. He sang his favorites from music therapy group – *BINGO, Wheels on the Bus, The Alphabet Song.* Then he sang a song I didn't even know he knew: *I Believe I Can Fly* (Kelly 1996). I'd known this boy for two years and had never heard him sing this song before, or request it in the music therapy group. This song also has special significance for me. Once I came upon one of my favorite patients singing it in his bed while watching the movie. This eight-year-old had been injured when he ran out in front of a car and was now a quadriplegic who was dependent upon a ventilator to breathe. Hearing a quadriplegic child sing *I Believe I Can Fly* can reduce me to a puddle of tears pretty darn fast. So I already have a history with this song.

Back at the bus stop, Andy finished singing and we called his dad back over to play it for him. When the tape progressed to that song, both his dad and I looked at each other and realized maybe something else was going on here. In fact, his dad quietly said to me, "I wonder if he's trying to tell me something." This child had relapsed twice with leukemia. I felt it likely that Andy might be trying to prepare his dad for his death in this non-threatening way.

We returned to the hospital and, of course, Andy insisted on playing his tape for all of his nurses, focusing on that one song. The more I heard it, the more it started getting to me. His doctors came into the room to examine him, and Andy played it for them. I excused myself under the ruse of privacy but mostly because by this time I was beginning to break down. Andy insisted that I remain right outside his open door, which I promised to do. Then he bellowed, "I can't see you!" I started waving my arm in the doorway and yelled, "I'm right here!" But of course, by this time I was crying. There I was, standing in the hallway, crying, and flapping one arm up and down in the doorway. One of our Child Life specialists walked by at that point and asked, "What are you doing?" I desperately said, "Just get me a tissue, please!"

It can be much easier to communicate in metaphor and song when you're a child with limited options.

Worst ages/best ages

There are some ages that are better than others for the various aspects of hospitalization. Toddlers are the worst age to have an IV pole. They love to walk, and they just don't get the fact that they're tethered to a pole. So they keep bolting away from it. Of course, the last thing we want is to lose the IV site, so parents, volunteers, and staff spend significant amounts of time lunging after toddlers who are running away from their IV poles.

Three-year-olds are the worst possible age to be stuck in isolation. They are social, they love the playroom and the music therapy group, and there is no way you can convince them of the need to stay in their rooms. They don't understand germs at all, and they feel they're the victims of a cruel conspiracy to deny them the pleasures of the playroom. They'll need a lot of one-to-one interaction in their rooms, and their parents will need a break!

Nine-year-old boys are the worst to be stuck in traction for broken legs. Unfortunately it seems that kids younger than nine can get a spica cast and go home; kids older than nine can be surgically pinned and go home. But nine-year-olds, because of their growth plates, (and I believe a sadistic tendency on the part of orthopedists – affectionately called "orthopods"), must be in the hospital, in traction, in their beds for at least six weeks. Traction is horrible for anybody, but it's especially bad for kids. Children need to move. My own observations lead me to believe that boys, in particular, interpret their world by bouncing off of it. To confine them to a bed with their leg swinging from weights in traction is not anyone's idea of a good time.

We deal with kids in long-term traction by bringing them (in bed) down to the playroom as soon as they're able to stand the trip. Keep in mind that in skeletal traction a child will have a large metal pin going through his bone that is attached by rope to weights hanging off the end of the bed. You will see this pin because it sticks out on either side of the leg. It looks terribly uncomfortable, and just a little bit "Frankensteinesque". Even with the most careful and experienced bed movers, and taping the rope to the bed frame with hospital-grade duct tape, those weights are going to swing a bit. And, of course, there are bumps going from linoleum to carpet in the playroom. What may seem like small, insignificant bumps to an ambulatory person are magnified about four million times to a child in traction. So we bring a lot of activities to the bedside until the wound has healed enough for the child to stand the movement of the bed. It's hard to believe, but the child soon habituates to the pin and the traction, and then moving the bed to the playroom is the easiest thing in the world. These kids almost always prefer to spend their days in the playroom, being included in all the activities, than being stuck in their rooms.

There is one age combination that I've found to be absolutely wonderful, and that is teenagers and guided imagery. This may be a reflection of my own ineptitude, or a result of their concrete style of thinking, but I've found it difficult to distract ten to twelve-year-olds with guided imagery, especially during painful procedures. For me, that age group is full of "Doubting Thomases". They look at me like I'm nuts. (Actually, I get that look a lot – but mostly in the music therapy group.) They're convinced they'll still feel pain, thereby negating all the positive effects that may have been generated by guided imagery.

Teenagers, however, seem to me to be the age group most open to guided imagery. This is particularly true for teens facing cancer – they are willing to try anything. I have taught guided imagery exercises to distract teenagers from painful procedures, for relaxation during bone marrow transplant, and have made custom tapes that help them get to sleep at night. (Teens tend to put on a brave face all day long, but in the wee hours of the morning their mortality can come crashing through and overwhelm them.) I've done guided imagery with kids as they lay dying in the hospital. That has been extremely satisfying for both the family and for me. Having an established relationship with the patient and the family has allowed me access into this private realm during the last days of a child's life.

I need to specify that I use a very simplified form of guided imagery. I am not trained in Helen Bonny's GIM (Guided Imagery with Music), but I am comfortable using soothing music with ocean sounds and giving suggestions for relaxation to a patient. I also count on the social worker to screen patients for me prior to a trial of guided imagery – kids with significant mental illness, and a loose hold on reality, would not be good candidates for me. And I always talk with the parents beforehand and get their permission.

Nicole

In my early days on Pediatrics, I met a ten-year-old girl and her mom who had been dealing with cancer for a few years. Nicole had rhabdomyosarcoma, a tumor that had started in her thigh muscle but metastasized. The cancer had unfortunately become resistant to treatment. Nicole and I began our relationship over keyboard lessons. I taught her simple tunes while her mother read a magazine nearby. Nicole's mom reminded me of a border collie – always watchful, never trusting. Periodically, her mom would make a comment that, while not exactly intimidating, was not quite supportive. She had raised her family by herself on a farm several hours away, and her daughter wasn't getting any better. Both mother and daughter seemed like private, reserved people who did not share anything of themselves and didn't expect much from the hospital staff.

One day the oncologist suggested I try guided imagery with Nicole, as the medical team had run out of options in fighting her cancer. I met Nicole's mom in the hallway to explain what guided imagery was and to ask her permission. As soon as she looked at me she said, "So, you're the last ditch" (as in "last ditch effort"). She agreed to let me try guided imagery with Nicole and went into her room with me. I explained guided imagery to Nicole and answered questions for both mother and daughter. As I got the tape recorder ready, Nicole's mother said, "Well, I'll let you two alone to work on this," and she left the room. I was amazed. This woman had never shown any trust to me before, and here she was leaving me alone with her daughter. She may have been desperate to find something that might help Nicole and wanted her to be able to concentrate fully on the imagery without the distraction of her mother in the room.

Nicole was the exception to my "ten-year-olds don't trust guided imagery" problem. She was very compliant with my requests for deep breathing and closing her eyes. She seemed like a good candidate for imagining her white blood cells going on the attack against tumor cells. Although Nicole and I had worked together for several hospital admits by this point, our relationship was not the head-over-heels love affair that I've experienced with many other kids. But there was a quiet, reserved friendship between us.

Nicole was out of the hospital for many months. I kept tabs on the family via the social worker. They were all apparently enjoying the summer together – doing lots of swimming, and having fun.

I had a dream about Nicole. In the dream, we had arranged that she would take the bus down to Sacramento and we would go out to lunch together. When I met her at the bus, a crocodile followed her down the steps. It followed us down the sidewalk, and into the restaurant. I stared at this crocodile, but Nicole didn't seem to notice it. At one point, I said, "Nicole, there's a crocodile following you." But she didn't say anything. She simply ignored it. When I woke up, I realized the crocodile was her cancer, closing in.

The next day Nicole was in the hospital, dying. In rounds, the nurse advised us to go in and say goodbye to her. The medical staff felt she had a few more hours to live. The patient's room was full of family members, but they let me come in. Nicole by this point looked more like an alien than the girl I knew and dreamt about. Her head seemed larger than her frail body. She was unresponsive and slowly ebbing away.

I kissed her head and started talking to her. Her mother indicated that she felt Nicole was lingering for some reason, and she was anxious that Nicole not suffer for any longer than necessary. I asked if I could try some guided imagery with Nicole again, to perhaps ease her mind and her transition. She agreed. I put my hand around Nicole's hand, and got very close to her ear. I told my friend about a book I'd read about people who had been resuscitated after being pronounced clinically dead. They'd shared very similar experiences – a feeling of love and warmth, beautiful meadows and flowers, friends who came to meet them, and absolutely nothing to be afraid of. Most of them didn't want to come back to life and leave this beautiful place. I also told Nicole that she was so important to all of us, especially her family. But the cancer was here to stay, and it wasn't going to let go. I told her that we would love her forever, and that she would be with us forever, and that no one in that room would ever forget her. I told her that it was OK for her to go, that her family would find a way to go on. I felt her finger move inside my hand.

Later in the day, I met Nicole's mom in the pantry. She was grateful for the imagery with Nicole and agreed that the only way she could communicate now was by barely moving her finger. The mom told me that their summer had been wonderful. Nicole had noticed that she was out of breath more and more, and her mom had tried to explain it was because of the cancer going into her lungs. Nicole hadn't brought it up again. I told her mom about my dream.

Nicole lived for three more days. Each day I went in to do guided imagery with her. The family held vigil around her bed but parted when I came in. One day, Mom was holding Nicole in a chair when I went in.

Mom said quite frankly, "I don't know why she's hanging on." She had asked all of her family members to tell Nicole directly that it was OK for her to die. This is frequently very effective. I told her that Nicole would go when she was ready, but in the meantime, it was nice to be able to hold her for this time. We did more imagery of a beautiful place to go, nothing to fear, and trusting that her family would always love her, would miss her, but would be able to go on. Nicole died that night.

The funeral was a three-hour drive away, and since I had a six-month old baby at home, I was unable to attend. I wrote a letter to Nicole's mom. Months later I got a Christmas card from Nicole's family. It was a photo of the family – mom and her two older children, with a small picture of Nicole included in the corner, "in memory". The mother had written a note to me all over the back of the card, but the first line was, "I will never forget you." Sometimes guided imagery will do as much for the family as for the patient.

Back door approach

I find that I have a back door approach to children who may be terrified and traumatized in a hospital. It seems as if the doctors and nurses come banging on the front door of a child and family and force their way in. I prefer the metaphor of going around the back and knocking quietly – just to see if anybody's home.

Sometimes it'll just happen that I'm working with a long-time patient who is the roommate of a scared new patient. The new child will see me laughing and making silly noises with her roommate and might show some interest in joining us. I have lots of keyboards, so I always offer one to the new patient and it becomes an easy, non-threatening way to start a relationship.

Sometimes a scared little one will be in the playroom for the first time. These are the times when I hope for a small, fairly quiet music therapy group, so the new child won't flip out and bolt. I've had kids who were too scared to join the group on their first day, but over the course of a week, they've moved closer and closer to the table loaded with instruments. Finally, and it may take a few days, or even a few admissions, the child will feel safe enough to join us and participate fully.

Ashley

One of my patients was a little three-year-old girl with AIDS who was the size of an undernourished one-year-old. Ashley was frail, lonely, terrified, and very sick. Her grandmother (the primary caretaker) was at home caring for her son, the little girl's father, who was actively dying of AIDS. It was a truly tragic family. As this little girl felt better, her nurse brought her to the music therapy group in a wagon. Ashley was so afraid of the other kids and all the new grown-ups, including me, that she cried if I even made eye contact with her from across the room (she was a "Don't look at me" kid). So I would look at every patient in my group and quickly look past her! This child would also cry if an instrument were offered to her.

Over the course of several days, Ashley gradually allowed me to look at her during group. Then I could smile at her. Then she would smile at me. She slowly evolved to the point where her wagon could be moved closer to the group, and she even accepted an instrument. She was so weak that she could only hold my lightest-weight bells or miniature maraca, but she would shake it for the duration of the song. She would grow tired of the effort of shaking and then shift the instrument from one hand to the other. She finally had to hold it with both hands. When she grew too tired to hold it, she'd drop it but continue to tap her hand on the side of the wagon. Some part of Ashley always had to keep the beat.

As she grew physically stronger, Ashley would move her whole body to the music. By this point, we had become very close friends, and she would become nearly ecstatic when I walked into the playroom for group. Then, unfortunately one of her visitors exposed her to chicken pox and she had to go into isolation. That was horrible – a three-year-old in isolation! Aaaagh! To make it even worse, she was isolated in the room next door to the playroom so she could hear us but not join us.

Every day, I'd take a few easy-to-clean instruments – Ashley was playing drums by now – and my guitar into her room 30 minutes before music therapy group started, and we'd have our own session. When I'd open the door, she'd get so excited that she'd shake her whole body back and forth and actually move the crib! This little girl was nonverbal but did try to sing and made various noises. I believe her delay may have been a function of her disease. I'd always arrange for a playroom volunteer to come into her room at 11:30 each day so I could leave to do the group, and my girl wouldn't be left alone. But Ashley figured that strategy out early on, and whenever a volunteer even opened the door, she'd start to cry. The only time she didn't cry was when her grandma was visiting. She loved her grandma.

It's not a wonderful thing to have to leave a crying three-year-old who desperately wants you to stay. Two-year-olds have done that to me on the burn unit, too. I like to leave kids laughing, not crying. But toddlers are very demonstrative in wanting to get you to stay. I just know the nurses are thinking, "Gee, thanks for your help, Kathy – now my kid's crying!" Sometimes I wonder if I should even go into a room if I know the patient will cry when I leave. My friends tell me, "It's better to have loved and lost, etc.", but it's hard, that's all I can say. Sometimes I can arrange to get another daily staff person, like the art therapist or a Child Life specialist to come in so the transition isn't so hard.

When Ashley was out of isolation and back in the playroom, we were once again a happy Pediatric floor. Soon she was well enough for discharge. She went home for a month, during which time her father died. Then she came back in with pneumonia and ended up on a ventilator in the PICU. I met her grandmother in the waiting room outside the unit and she told me about the death of her son, and how she and Ashley had had some wonderful time alone together. I had enormous regard for this woman. We had also grown close. I couldn't even begin to imagine the magnitude of her recent loss and the loss she would soon experience with her granddaughter.

Ashley deteriorated quickly. When I saw her in the PICU, I didn't even recognize her. My tiny little girl had swelled up tremendously, and tape covered most of her face where the breathing tube went into her mouth. She was heavily sedated, but I sang to her and told her goodbye. Saying goodbye to favorite patients is extremely important. When you get one more chance to say what you need to say, even though it's sad, it's so satisfying. It seals your relationship forever. One thing I've realized from losing so many children I've loved – the love never dies. The relationship is still alive, although the other person is no longer around. You still love them. Ashley died that night.

7. Welcome
to the Broken
Hearts Club

Friends

I wrote an article for Music Therapy Perspectives that was originally titled, "Friends: Death of a Favorite Patient." One of the editors suggested that I was opening myself up to criticism by using the word "friends". Within the article I had made mention of the fact that our hospital staff has been introduced by parents at funerals as "My hospital family", and the editor had no problem with that. But somehow we are not to be friends with our clients – that is crossing into dangerous waters.

I agree with that philosophy for virtually every other population music therapists work with: psychiatric, sexual offenders, substance abusers. Actually the other two populations with whom I've worked – developmentally delayed adults and geriatrics – were pretty lovable, too. But we're talking about kids, here and, somehow, our hospital gets the most beautiful kids in the world. Anyone who works with oncology patients knows that only the best people get cancer – kids and adults. It is an honor to work with them, and it is pretty danged hard not to fall in love with them.

Before I began working on Pediatrics, I believed in the myth of health care professionals remaining distant and aloof from their patients, so they wouldn't get hurt if the patient died. Well, having worked on Pediatrics for a long time, I can say that at least on our floor, that is a complete myth! It has no basis in reality at all. The truth is that we all get involved with these kids – it's virtually impossible to avoid. Kids just get to you. They give you a smile or a hug, and you can feel yourself becoming completely wrapped around their little bitty fingers. They know what they're doing, you know what they're doing, but you're powerless against them.

I've heard it's a tenet of evolution – that baby animals are cute so that the adults will become bonded and provide them with the best possible care. It's supposed to ensure the survival of the species. It surely works at our hospital. There is also a basic tenet of nursing – nurturing creates bonding. When you take care of someone, you become connected to that person. They become important to you.

I know the arguments for remaining "professional" and aloof from your clients. In my sixteen years of working on Pediatrics, I have seen only two instances of what I would consider to be inappropriate bonding. In both cases the health care worker was a single woman who insinuated herself into the family as if it were her own. One of these people, a home health nurse, was so intrusive and opinionated that I believe it had a negative impact on the family's grieving the loss of their son.

It is important to remember that our needs are not our patients' needs. Their needs come first – our needs come last, at home. Our homes. However, if you work with seriously ill children, you're going to lose part of your heart to them, and it will be extremely painful when they die. You're not going to avoid it.

This means that if you suffer from chronic depression, or are carrying around unresolved grief, this is probably not the ideal population for you. It is also helpful if your family situation is stable. I know that life is messy and gets in the way of a lot of things, but if my home life is in upheaval, I simply don't have the wherewithal to deal with the emotional demands of my job. Pediatrics can be a hard place to work. I am constantly aware that my coworkers are among the bravest people in the world. They are willing to go into the room of a child with a terrible prognosis and offer the family friendship and help at the worst point in their lives.

The people who can't handle this find other jobs. Three years seem to be a cut-off point for a lot of staff. While it is important to have consistent staff daily, it is also critical to have long-term staff. Oncology patients may relapse, and kids with sickle cell anemia and cystic fibrosis will be hospitalized repeatedly over the course of their lives. These patients especially need to see a familiar face when they return.

The children who are frequently admitted are obviously the ones we get to know best. We work with them over the course of years, and we develop close relationships with the kids and their families. The patients themselves seem to take comfort from these friendships and will boast to our college volunteers, "Kathy's known me since I was a baby." Sometimes they will compete with each other over how long they've known us. "Oh yeah? Well, she's known me for 12 years. Beat that!"

Boundaries

I define emotional boundaries as a set of rules that a health care worker establishes for herself. As music therapists, we can refer to the American Music Therapy Association Code of Ethics and the Standards of Practice, but ultimately we are responsible for setting our own boundaries in working with patients. One interesting aspect to boundary setting is that what may seem comfortable to one person will inevitably be judged by everyone else, i.e., "That nurse has no boundaries!" Some of our nurses have gone to Disneyland with their patients for Make-A-Wish.[1] Some go to concerts, or skiing with their patients when they're out of the hospital. We had a foster grandpa who was so popular with the kids that he was frequently invited to their birthday parties outside the hospital. Conversely I know of a Child Life program in a children's hospital that forbids their staff from attending funerals of patients – for them that is crossing the line.

It is important to establish your own boundaries. Some of my rules include:

1. I don't give money to patients.

2. I don't bring my kids to the hospital.

3. I don't take time away from my kids to be with my patients, i.e., I rarely attend weekend funerals.

4. Time away from my patients is okay, i.e., lunch, vacations.

---

[1] Make-A-Wish is a wonderful non-profit organization that grants wishes to kids with terrible diseases. Kids have met celebrities, gone to Disneyland and Disney World, been given computers, etc.

Now, of course, I have broken every single one of these rules in my pediatric career, but each time before I do, my rule looms up large in my face so that I examine it carefully before I break it. It is a rule, after all – and one that I set up, myself. For instance, although I do not give money to patients, I have bought a pizza for a child in bone marrow transplant. And I happily donate to graduation and birthday gifts, and funeral expenses for financially strapped patients of mine.

I had a serious conflict once when the funeral of a favorite patient coincided with a cross-country ski trip I had planned with my own family. I had loved the child, and loved her mother, and felt deeply that I needed to be at that funeral. My own kids are very understanding about my work, and they were even supportive of my attending the funeral. That rule bothered me for several days before I finally made the decision to be with life rather than death that day. I still feel that I made the right decision, but I will always feel guilty that I missed that funeral. Writing a card to the mother just didn't fill that need.

Once the art therapist asked our supervisor for permission to bring her daughter to the floor on the weekend so that she could visit one of her patients. Her daughter and this patient shared the same first name, and she thought it would be fun to introduce them. Our supervisor thought it would be fine and they had a great little visit. It struck me because one of my rules is that I don't like to mix my home life with my hospital life. Many of our nurses bring their new babies to the floor, something I have never done. Mostly I am concerned with germs. The hospital is a green-house full of germs – why would I want to expose my kids to that? Also, my kids may have been exposed to some evil virus and not show symptoms but may still be contagious. I would not want to share that with one of my immune-suppressed patients. There have been occasions, however, when I've been asked to perform for the Oncology Christmas party at night, or the Cardiac Surgery Reunion on a Saturday, in which case I've brought my kids. They've been handy in hauling instruments from the playroom to wherever the party was, but we've never visited patients while we've been there.

Recently I broke another rule. Lunchtime is sacred to me – a chance to be away from the kids for 45 minutes, and chat with the grown-ups. I learn a lot from the nurses, we laugh a lot. Lunch is my time. But I had a little five-year-old girl with Wilm's tumor (a kidney tumor) whose family just couldn't make it to the hospital. The mother had three other kids at home and car problems. The father was in jail. The problem was that the mother would frequently promise Annie that she'd be in soon and bring something special when she came, like Chinese food. The mother constantly broke her promises and the little girl was desperately lonely. She would attend my music therapy group and then ask me to walk her back to her room. Then when I tried to leave, she would cling to me, and we faced the recurrent dance of trying to peel her off me and interest her in lunch. I tried to get volunteers to stay with her, but she threw them out of her room. On the weekends she ate lunch at the nurses' station, but that was lonely, too, since half the nurses were in the report room eating lunch and the remainder were busy with patients.

I finally realized that it was more traumatic for both of us to uphold my rule of lunchtime is my time. I told Annie, "Let's make a deal. If you're here at the hospital, and I'm here at the hospital, we'll have lunch together." She was amazed. Everyday she asked me, "Please, Kathy, please will you have lunch with me today?" Everyday we ate together. She was just a kid who needed more than a half-hour intervention of music therapy. She needed a consistent adult in her life. An amazing development occurred after we started having lunch together – Annie became more willing to go with other staff members and volunteers. After we finished lunch, she didn't need me anymore. Now it may have been just coincidence, or her getting used to the hospital routine and environment, but the timing was so immediate that I have to believe our lunches had something to do with it.

Giving up my private lunchtime was a big commitment to this little girl. She had cancer – she would be coming in frequently for chemotherapy and for fevers and low blood counts. Again my rule loomed in my face demanding I examine this situation. So I did examine it, then I broke it, and I committed my lunchtimes to this little girl whenever she was admitted. An interesting phenomenon came up as a result of my lunchtimes with Annie – the nurses were extremely grateful, but some newer staff members complained, "Kathy has no boundaries!"

An important thing to remember is that you don't work in a void. At lunchtime, ask the nurses for their opinions on boundaries. Talk to people who have been in the profession for a few years, rather than new graduates. Get together with other therapists who work in similar settings. Above all, when setting your boundaries think or write your way through the process – don't react impulsively or from guilt. If you respect your boundaries, others will, too.

Psychosocial aspects to cancer

When a child is diagnosed with cancer, the world changes drastically for the family. They spend the first admission to the hospital – the work-up and diagnosis – in a state of shock mixed with a large dose of terror. There is no one on the planet as precious as a child, and when one is threatened, a parent's world falls apart. But the parents I work with heroically try to hold it together so their child doesn't become even more scared. The level of stress that parents and children live through after an initial diagnosis of cancer is staggering.

A music therapist needs to be very sensitive to the stress roiling about in the room at this time. Sometimes the child screams at one more person entering, wrongly assuming you're bringing more pain. It's hard to communicate to parents over the screams of their child, so at these times I just hold up the keyboard and try to mouth – "I'll be back later." I'll ask the nurse to be sure to let the family know about our music therapy group, and when they're ready, I'll be available. Again, the kid sees me leave, feels the power of throwing me out, but also saw the keyboard. I'll be back later in the afternoon, or the next day. Maybe the family will be in the playroom later, and we can play together there.

Once you build a relationship with a scared child, you almost automatically earn the trust of the parents. If you make their child laugh, you earn intense gratitude. Parents will see you as important to their child's well being while hospitalized, and by extension, their own. Parents will seek you out to vent emotions – frustration, anger, fear – because they trust you. Frequently parents are afraid to vent their feelings to medical or nursing staff. They worry that it may adversely affect the care of their child. So they'll single you out in the playroom, or they'll stop you in the hallway, or they'll meet you at the bus stop to talk. It's important for parents to be able to vent frustration, and it's easy for us to listen. After all, they're not complaining about us, and we can find the right person to help the situation.

After the first hospitalization, when everything is weird, alien and often painful for the child and the parents are as stressed as they're ever going to be in their lives, the next admission will be easier. Kids are usually pretty good about adjusting to the new environment. Once they discover the playroom and the music therapy group – the normal parts of the hospital – they feel more at home. It is essential that the child doesn't live in dread of the hospital, especially if it is going to be part of their lives for a while.

Once I was playing with a three-year-old in the playroom, and her mother recounted how, the night before, she'd try to prepare her daughter for returning to the hospital the next day for chemotherapy. The girl immediately threw a huge fit. Finally the mom realized that her daughter wanted to come to the hospital *that night!* She didn't want to wait until the next day. This is not a frequent occurrence – we don't get a lot of kids banging on the doors and begging to come in. But this episode let me know we're doing something right.

Being willing to extend ourselves to these families at the most devastating point in their lives can form rather deep relationships. We're walking on holy ground here. We'll see these families repeatedly over the next six months for inpatient chemotherapy. They'll frequently drop by after that for visits when they have clinic appointments. Then anytime the child develops a fever, or is exposed to chicken pox, she will be admitted. Sometimes we'll see these families at the funerals of other kids, because the cancer families often form strong support systems among each other. All of these contacts build upon the layers of relationship/friendship/extended family feeling between hospital staff and families.

Bad times – relapse

Relapse is just about the worst thing that can happen to a child with cancer and his family. He's already been through this. He did everything the doctors told him to do. He did his best, he put up with the hair loss, the vomiting, etc., and the cancer still came back. He knows he has to go through it all over again. It is a desperate time for all, but it makes a difference having staff around that the family has known from before. These are the folks the parents don't have to explain anything to, because we already understand. The important thing now is to find a way to accept this new setback and move on.

Once a child relapses, the chance for recovery narrows. The doctors gave the best medicines for remission the first time around, and on each relapse (there can be many) they bring out bigger guns. Harsher, more toxic medicines have more severe side effects. It can get to the point where the chemotherapy may destroy the cancer, but may actually kill the child in the process. You can imagine the stress and hopelessness parents would be fighting at this point. They need all the support they can get. Sometimes even their friends and family from outside the hospital are too much for them to deal with, because they get tired of explaining the same thing to everyone over and over. They need people to just understand and help with their child.

When a patient is diagnosed as terminally ill and has a code of DNR (Do Not Resuscitate), he starts to shut down on extraneous relationships. We frequently put up signs on the door, at the patient's request, that read, "No new staff." This is another reason why it's important to have long-term folks around.

When a child is dying in the hospital, the doctors and nurses are especially attuned. We try to get the family one of the large, private rooms. Sometimes another bed is moved in for the parents' use. Earlier in the process, the doctors will talk with the parents, and the patient if she's a teenager, about the future prospects. Since current fear of litigation demands that medical staff resuscitate anyone who stops breathing, they need a DNR order in the front of the chart if the family so wishes. The worst-case scenario occurs when a dying child has no such order, is resuscitated by CPR (cardiopulmonary resuscitation) and ends up on a ventilator in the PICU. This is where the vent is the only thing keeping the child alive. As hard as it is to watch a child die, removing him from the vent is even worse. Plus, the family is in the PICU with all new nursing staff and a lot more rules on how many people can be in the room at a time, and restricted times when the parents have to leave the unit.

Sometimes kids have slipped past us. They've been transferred from their community hospital where they were treated too long and too ineffectively for an infection that has taken over. By the time they're sent to us, the infection is systemic and hopelessly entrenched. They end up on a vent in the PICU.

If this happens to one of my patients from music therapy group, I'll go to the PICU and sing to them. They know my voice, they know the songs, and it's a way of continuing our relationship. It's also a way of saying goodbye. The family appreciates the connection. Sometimes we sing together to their child – that can be truly beautiful and extremely therapeutic for all of us.

Pediatrics is a different realm. It's hard to go through years of contact with families, with their children smiling and laughing at you, running down the hall to hug you, or yelling at you to come see them, without getting more than just a tad involved. There have been kids who I truly didn't know if I could survive losing. In talking with our nurses and Child Life folks, we all agree that we are closer to some of these families than we are to our own extended families. We are honored to participate in this sacred, caregiving relationship. It opens our hearts and expands our souls. If "friends" is not an acceptable word to use, then help me come up with another.

Father and son

I recently heard from a single dad who lost his six-year-old son to leukemia within the past year. We'd worked with these two guys for two and a half years. His son's last admission was supposed to be for four days of scheduled chemotherapy in April. It stretched until November when he died. Over the course of those long months, the dad grew to trust several of us. He even referred to us as his sisters. The last hospitalization included open-heart surgery to remove calcification caused by the broviac catheter, neuropathy (a side effect of chemotherapy that left Bobby with paralyzed lower extremities, weakened upper extremities, and pain throughout), and pneumonia. Bobby regained arm function following the neuropathy, but he was never able to use his legs again. He was transferred to the inpatient rehabilitation service to help him deal with his newly acquired paraplegia and to rebuild his strength.

There was the on again/off again promise of a bone marrow transplant at another hospital, but he had to be in remission, well enough and strong enough to survive the intense levels of chemotherapy and radiation involved. When he was finally ready, the donor was on vacation and unavailable! That window was soon shut forever.

At one point in this boy's stay, I was seeing him twice/day, for music therapy/fun, and to be his support person during physical therapy and occupational therapy, which were quite difficult for him. His dad, who was always at the bedside, couldn't stand watching his boy in pain and would ask me to stay while he left for a cigarette break during that time.

Over the course of this long stay, the entire Pediatric floor pitched in to keep this boy occupied. One of his primary nurses brought in a flying toy bat that she hung from the ceiling. By pushing a button, we could get that bat to fly in a circle above Bobby's head. The medical students assigned to him rigged up a huge plastic spider with a long cord that reached from the TV to Bobby's hand. Bobby would innocently tell a newcomer that he was having problems with his TV, and could they reach up and turn it on for him? Then he would let go of his line and the spider would fall on top of the innocent bystander. It was always good for a laugh.

For Bobby's Make-A-Wish, he had practically bought out a toy store, so we had a lot of material to choose from in his room. He particularly enjoyed fighting with his wrestling models. One day while we were so engaged, he said, "Hey! Did you know these are really walkie-talkies?" Well, I'd wondered why they had holes in their bare chests, but that hadn't occurred to me. So we started talking into them to see if they worked. Soon he sent me out of his room into the hallway to get some distance between us. Bobby, from the safety of his bed, yelled, "Louder!" I, however, was out in the hallway being passed by doctors, nurses, families, housekeepers, and medical students, as I spoke commando dialogue into the naked chest of a wrestling model. (Remember that feedback I got from my presentation at the American Music Therapy Association National Conference where someone was annoyed that I don't do music therapy 100% of the time? She or he would've loved this!)

Bobby and three other boys who were also frequently hospitalized formed a strong support group among themselves. These boys coached each other through some terrible times of pain, loneliness, grief, and sudden and awful new developments in the course of their respective diseases. They found in each other hope, courage, and love. They touched all of us.

We all went through a lot of pain, terror, grief, joy, sadness, and silliness together. At one point I was walking down the hall with Bobby's dad while a nurse walked behind us. The dad said, "I need a Kathy hug." So I hugged him until he let go, and as I stepped away, the nurse behind me stepped forward and hugged him, too. I thought, "That's what's so good about this place. If you need a hug, you get two." We are a loving staff and we are helping families deal with horrendous issues.

I think half of the hospital staff attended this child's funeral. Although I wondered if there were any nurses on Pediatrics that day, it was important for the dad to see all of us there. Recently this dad told one of his son's primary nurses, "I felt more love at that hospital than at any other point in my life." That is desperately sad to me, but then I think – thank God he had that love when it was crucial for him.

We get close to families, and I truly believe that is OK.

We also get close to each other. There are many nurses who I call "Honey", or "Hon." But I'm old and can get away with it. I *never* call kids "Honey." Having lunch with the nurses gets us talking together. Going to funerals and grieving together bonds us. We all agree that we couldn't survive this setting without the constant support of each other. We cry together a lot. We need to talk to get these feelings out, but there are very few people outside the hospital who can bear to listen to stories of dying children. We understand and support each other. We are also extended family to each other. I hope we are not unique. I hope many hospitals have staff like this.

8. The Art
of the Family

Hospitalization as a monkey wrench

Anyone who works with the public knows what a challenge that can be. Add to that challenge the stress of diagnosing their children with a potentially fatal disease and you have the most difficult public you're ever going to meet! Even for families with chronically ill kids, who have been dealing with this for all of the child's life, hospitalization is a major inconvenience. Having a child in the hospital throws a very big monkey wrench into the machinery of the most well oiled family life.

A head nurse of the PICU once told me that on any given day, most of the families in her unit were crazy. She was serious. She felt they were mentally ill. I thought, "Honey, put one of *my* kids on this unit and you will see a *real* crazy parent!" Most of our staff members have kids of their own, and they know the raw terror of having something happen to their kids. Ironically, on the general pediatric floor, some of our most understanding nurses don't have kids of their own. But they love working with kids (and think adults smell bad!).

Although we, as hospital staff, may start thinking of the hospital as a normal place, it will never be anywhere close to normal for our patients and their families. Sometimes, particularly if the diagnosis is dire, there may be many horrible associations with the hospital. Even though we are very conscious of pain – it has become a fifth vital sign that nurses routinely check for – there is just no way around the fact that pain is a prevalent part of hospitalization. In fact, it can be easy for the majority of a parent's last memories of their child to be full of misery, pain, and discomfort. Terminal cancer can cause intractable pain that the most consci-entious oncologist and pain service doctors can find nearly impossible to treat.

So, pain and discomfort, boredom, terror – man, hospitals are terrible places! And certainly no place for a child! It is critical that these kids and families have something other than negative stimulation in a place like this. That's when I feel that part of my job is to be the Happiness Monitor. I try to set up opportunities for fun and positive interactions to occur between kids and their families.

One time I walked into a room as the doctors were walking out. They had just explained to the family that their beautiful two-year-old boy had relapsed and there was really nothing more they could do to treat his cancer. The family had been expecting this, but still it was horrible. The family realized, though, that their child was feeling pretty well at the moment, and regardless of what the future held, right now we had a little boy who wanted to play drums. I handed out percussion instruments to mom, dad, siblings and grandma, and we sang all of this boy's favorite songs. I will always remember this child as the one whose favorite animal for the farm songs was a mongoose! (And a mongoose sounds like? Rikki Tikki Tavi, of course. Let me tell you, that can really cramp up your tongue when you stick it on *Old McDonald's Farm*, but it's for a good cause and we can all laugh in the process.)

Another two-year-old buddy of mine was in the hospital a lot. He was a patient who was fairly difficult to reach. Sometimes he was feeling so lousy that he wanted nothing and just cried. But if he felt at all well enough, we played together. Somehow it's the kids who are the hardest to reach who become the most important to you. He had a very special smile. At one point, he and his mom and I were playing around on the Rapman keyboard on his bed. This keyboard came with a microphone that had various settings – it could make your voice sound high like you were playing with helium, or low like the Creature from the Black Lagoon. It was a wonderful keyboard.

Two-year-olds are great parrots, and they'll frequently mimic you. While we were being silly, I said into the microphone to this little boy, "I love you, mommy." He immediately took the microphone, smiled at her and said, "I love you, mommy." Mom, in turn, leaned into the mic and said, "I love you, Kevin," and they repeated this exchange over and over until they fell on top of each other, laughing. This is one of my favorite memories. This little boy died awaiting a bone marrow transplant at another hospital. When I heard the news I cried for two days. I simply couldn't stop crying. I couldn't even work for those two days. He was just one of those kids.

The important thing is to set up opportunities for families to have a wonderful time being a family together. Then we step back and let the family members do the important work. We have to have some good memories in this horrendous environment. The families need them. I need them.

Siblings

Since Pediatrics is the art of working with families, siblings frequently play a large role at our hospital. Brothers and sisters, cousins, etc. come to the playroom nearly as often as the patients. There have been times when my music therapy group has been entirely made up of siblings. I give siblings the same amount of love and care that I extend to my patients. They are frequently struggling with many issues when their brother or sister is hospitalized.

Siblings don't understand why their parents are treating the patient so nicely all of a sudden. They're jealous that the patient gets gifts when they get nothing. Siblings have been overheard to say, "I wish I had leukemia." They tend to only see the positive side of hospitalization, not the pain and fear involved. Parents are barely able to deal with the needs of their hospitalized child and have little or no energy left for the well children. Parents may expect the other children to behave in a more mature and understanding fashion, which is unrealistic. Siblings glean most of their information from overhearing whispered parental conversations in the hallway. This is almost never accurate and can be easily distorted by a child's imagination. They are also very afraid for their brother or sister but feel they cannot bring this fear to their parents. Siblings get a raw deal whenever a child is hospitalized.

Siblings need support, too. They need someone to listen to them, to play with them, to make them feel special and appreciated. They need someone to get them away from the sick child and parents when things become chaotic and the parents' fuse is ready to detonate. Siblings need relationships with hospital staff just as much as the patients and parents.

Siblings are also a resource. They may be willing to participate with you before the sick and scared child is ready. Siblings have gotten my foot in the door of an otherwise terrified patient. The sick child will see me interacting and having fun with their brother or sister and will cautiously ask to join us. Other times siblings have attended music therapy group on their own and reported back to the family. The next day I've had the entire family in the group. It's also very important for siblings of children in the PICU to be able to hang out in the playroom. These kids need normalcy more than anyone. They can only tolerate the stress of the PICU for limited periods before becoming a very big problem for the parents, who are already at the brink.

Brothers

One day I noticed two very healthy looking boys in the playroom before I went over to the PICU for rounds. In the meeting I learned that these boys were the brothers of a baby who was dying in the PICU. This baby was six months old and had been born with a terrible skin problem that constantly looked like a third degree (now called full thickness) burn. This infant had endured chronic infections and pain throughout his short life, and his single mother decided he had been through enough. We had never seen this baby before – another hospital had transferred him to us. The mother was much better informed on this rare disease than any of our doctors, and they respected her wishes. She'd talked with her older sons (ages eight and ten) about the baby's condition, and now they were in the playroom. Apparently the older boy wanted to be at the baby's bedside if possible at the moment of death, but the younger one didn't.

When I returned to the playroom, the volunteers informed me that the two boys had been very verbal about their baby's dying. This was an amazing family. Rarely do we see parents and children who are so open with each other about the subject of death. At the moment, however, the boys and another male patient (aged 12) were locked in a yelling battle over a board game. "You cheater!" "Who are you calling cheater, cheater?" The patient stood up, ready to storm out of the playroom in an angry huff. I got the drums out and tried to create a new atmosphere quickly. "Don't leave, Titus. I need you to show these guys how to play my drums." He sat back down, and the boys watched in amazement as I pulled drums out for them to play. We fell into a structured improvization, each of the kids taking turns leading the group, the rest watching and listening carefully so that they could imitate and follow. The boys loved the drums and a feeling of cooperation was born among the kids. When the group was playing together, in a groove, it was an amazing feeling – very satisfying on an internal level. It was a beautiful feeling of "flow". When we didn't quite get there, it felt very disjointed. We became adept at listening to each other. These kids were now smiling who had been screaming at each other just a few minutes before.

Toward the end of our group, a woman came to the doorway of the playroom and motioned for the boys to come with her. The boys didn't want to stop drumming, so I stopped the group and the woman said, "It's time." The oldest son asked, "Are they cutting him loose?" She nodded tearfully, and both boys sprang up and bolted to the door. The youngest turned back to us and said, "We'll be back!" I was absolutely struck by the phrase the ten-year-old used – "Cutting him loose." It sounded so positive, like a kite with a string that's caught and tugging in the wind to be set free. I had no worries about this family. I knew they would be just fine.

Brandy

Another time I had an 11-year-old sibling in music therapy group whose younger sister was dying of Wilm's tumor (a tumor that starts on the kidney). For days their hospital room had been packed with family and friends keeping vigil at the bedside. These two girls were the only children in the family and they'd been very close, but this sister needed a break from the deathbed and joined us. In the middle of the group, a family member came rushing down to the playroom and tapped this girl on the shoulder. She left with her aunt, and then minutes later came running back to the music therapy group. She stood in the middle of the playroom. I stopped the group and asked, "Brandy?" She blurted out, "She's gone!" I said, "Oh, Brandy, I'm so sorry." She came over to me and I put my arm around her as she cried. Of course, one of the kids in the group asked, "Where'd she go?" I gently explained to this group of all ages of children that Brandy's sister had just died. They asked, "What did she die of?" Brandy told them, "Cancer." At this point another family member came to the playroom to retrieve and comfort Brandy. Since nearly all of my groups have at least one oncology patient in them, I explained that there are many different types of cancer, and we have very strong medicines that fight them. However, in this case, Brandy's sister had a very bad cancer that was too strong for our medicine. I was able to tell the children with cancer in my group specifically that they had a different type of cancer and that they would be all right. It was an intense group situation, but I was struck by Brandy's need to tell us in the music therapy group about her sister's death. Perhaps it was just that she needed to tell somebody, or it might have been that the group was a source of support for her. It was quite striking how she fled her sister's room, where her extended family was, and came running to us. Siblings need support.

Funerals

I go to enough funerals to qualify as a regular church-goer. There are times when I think I've gone to every church in Northern California. I don't like funerals – sometimes it's like walking into a migraine. And the sayings that get people through – "He had a long and productive life" – are completely irrelevant when it's for a two-year-old. The first time I saw a three-foot long casket, it overwhelmed me. Children are just not supposed to die.

When the music starts you realize everything you learned in school about music cutting past all the defenses and going straight to your heart is absolutely true. I take lots of tissues with me. Once I was sitting in the second row with two nurse friends behind the patient's dad. They were the patient's primary nurses, and I, of course, was his primary music therapist. We'd all become very close to this family. My nurse friend, who has small children at home, which automatically equals chaos, reached into her purse when she started crying. She pulled out a half-roll of toilet paper and whispered, "I was in a hurry and couldn't find anything else!" Luckily, I always take enough tissues for everyone, so we avoided that spectacle of her pulling out a length of toilet paper every time she blew her nose.

I go to funerals for a couple of reasons: to support the family, and for the catharsis of crying my eyes out. I discovered early in my years on

Pediatrics that if I can hug the family after the death, I can heal. Hugging the family somehow wraps up our relationship for me. It completes the circle. We have all gone through some profound times together, and it's crucial for me to be able to acknowledge that at the end. There are no words that are adequate, but then no words are necessary. What's important is that you just hold on.

At one funeral that I attended, I wondered if the mother would accept hugs. She'd been fairly difficult and distant from the staff during her five-year-old son's illness, and had horrendous problems with her husband. Before the funeral began, while the huge audience slowly filed in and found seats, and the organ solemnly played, this mother jumped up whenever she saw people she knew and literally ran to hug them. Her need was so great that she simply couldn't sit still. She desperately held onto the people she needed to get her through this.

I lost a four-year-old buddy during bone marrow transplant at another hospital. I'd known him and his mom for three years. I couldn't get to the funeral due to babysitter problems. I felt a huge open wound in my heart from not seeing the mom after his death. I called her on the phone and we talked for an hour, but that didn't heal me. I knew I had to see her. Unfortunately she lived 100 miles away, up in the mountains. Once I was headed up toward her town for my daughter's field trip, and wrote a letter suggesting we meet at the site of the field trip. But the letter came back. She had moved and I didn't have her new address or phone. One day, three years after her son's death, this mom stopped by the hospital. She stood crying outside the Child Life office – she couldn't even walk onto the Pediatric floor. The Child Life folks found me, and I was able to hug her and cry with her. From that point on, I was able to heal. I know that if she hadn't stopped by, or if I had been gone that day, I would still have an open wound inside my chest. It's very important for me to hug the families.

Sometimes I don't know the families. They visit their child in the evening when I'm gone, or they have transportation problems, or other kids at home. If that's the case, I don't need to attend the funeral. Open caskets do nothing for me. I'm often struck how little the shell resembles the life it used to be. I love photos that are on prominent display at funerals, because that's the kid I used to know and love.

I worry about families after their child dies. While the child is dying in the hospital, there is a lot of support. But then the child is gone, and the family leaves, and we stay at the hospital. The transition must be incredible. Sometimes their extended families are not reliable, and after the flurry of the funeral, their support evaporates. Our social workers keep tabs on our bereaved families, and the oncology parents have an extensive support group. I write to the families after a child's death. I try to resurrect one of my favorite memories to give to the parents. Once a dad requested that our staff write down favorite memories of his son in a journal he dropped off. Weeks earlier, when we'd learned that his son had relapsed, I'd gone home and written nine pages on this little guy for my own therapy. From that raw material I typed up three pages and sent it to the dad. He told me later that whenever he was down, he'd get that letter out and cry over it, and laugh over it.

I'm finding myself in a position now where I just call or write to parents who've been on my mind a lot. I figure that if they don't want to communicate, they'll let me know. But so far, the feedback has been very positive.

9. Critical Care Units

Pediatric Intensive Care Unit

To a child, the pediatric intensive care unit (PICU) must be as familiar as the cockpit of a space shuttle. There are so many beeps, clicks, hums and buzzes that alarm for every piece of machinery that it's like being in another world altogether. PICUs also have more rules regarding who can visit and when. Sometimes parents are not allowed to spend the night at the child's bedside.

Some intensive care units (ICUs) have the lights on 24 hours/day. The noisy alarms (causing sensory overload) combine with the complete lack of naturally occurring, familiar sounds (sensory deprivation). Any patient who is critically ill simply cannot interpret this overwhelming sensory input. Added to this scenario is sleep deprivation that is caused by frequent, even if necessary, interruptions by nursing staff. Then there is the noise level of the medical staff conferring over the bed. This has actually been measured to reach the decibel level of a Mack truck since they have to talk over the machinery and alarms. It is understandable how some patients actually begin to experience visual and auditory hallucinations, called ICU Psychosis. This delusional state usually clears up within 24 hours of a patient being moved to a general floor. If ICUs are this hard on adults, you can imagine how difficult it must be for a child. Patients may also be going through withdrawal from narcotics if they are not properly weaned from them. It can be hard to tell what's going on with little ones in the PICU.

So, ICUs can make you crazy. On top of that, parental stress is ratcheted up several notches because having your child in the PICU is just about as scary as it gets. Then, of course, someone in the next room may have stopped breathing, or may even be dying, and then a code to resuscitate is announced. This involves a lot of people, equipment, noise, upheaval, and stress, not only for the patient and family involved, but also for everyone else in the unit.

I am not afraid of death, but I am afraid of becoming a patient in the ICU. It can be depressing just to attend rounds in the PICU. The children are supremely sick or have barely survived terrible accidents. Many are on ventilators. Some may be actually brain dead, which entails its own medical protocol and tremendous stress for the family.

I follow kids I know from the general pediatric floor who may end up in the PICU due to sepsis (systemic bacterial infection) or other problems. I am also referred to patients who may be just waking up from coma or heavy sedation and who need positive and familiar types of stimulation.

If one of my patients needs to transfer from the general floor to the PICU, it's very important for me to continue the relationship, especially for the parents. They have new nurses who do not know their child. The child may be sedated and on a ventilator to help him avoid the sheer labor of breathing, and this is a terrifically scary time for parents. Bringing the normalcy of the child's favorite songs from the music therapy group to the PICU is normalizing for all of us. It also brings hope that this is just a temporary glitch in the healing process. Our support can also aid the family if this is a more permanent glitch and recovery is looking like less of an option. Our job is to listen and to support the family wherever they may be in the grieving process. Showing up daily, listening to the parents, offering a shoulder to cry on, or holding a hand is invaluable. Parents need all the love and support they can get at this point.

It's also wonderful to slowly begin a relationship with a new child in the PICU and then follow her to the general floor. I feel that's the true miracle of rehabilitation. The children come into the hospital and we meet them when they're sedated and on a vent. Then they're awake and barely interacting with us. Then suddenly it seems they're walking to music therapy group. And the next thing you know they're skipping down the hallway and we're all singing them the rehab goodbye song.

DJ

There was a time when I had a two-year-old man of my dreams for a series of long hospitalizations. This little boy was deaf and had AIDS, and we were in love. He was living with his aunt who was also raising five other kids. She was quite busy at home, therefore DJ was frequently in my arms whenever he was hospitalized. One time I walked past the nurses' station and didn't even notice DJ sitting there in his high chair, eating. But I heard his distinctive noisy yell at me. I stopped and waved, and the nurse who was feeding him said, "Kathy, what is it between you and DJ?" I said, "We have a 'thing' going on."

One day in the middle of a huge music therapy group, DJ decided to throw one of his world-class tantrums. I was in the middle of a song and tried to signal with my strumming hand to a new Child Life specialist to get DJ out of the group until he could calm down. Frequently it just takes someone holding a toddler, walking around and talking soothingly, and then they can come right back to group. Sometimes it takes more. Sometimes two-year-olds just need to scream it out for a while. However, it is fairly distracting when a two-year-old is melting down in the middle of a song. The Child Life specialist didn't pick up on my hand signals, but DJ did. He misinterpreted my "heave-ho" gesture, as "she wants me". Sobbing, he walked toward me with arms outstretched. I placed my guitar on the table and put DJ on my lap, whereupon he immediately stopped crying. I picked up my guitar (this is why God gave me long arms) and finished the group with DJ on my lap. And I thought – these kids constantly teach me new things. Never would I have dreamed that putting a screaming toddler on my lap during music therapy group would calm him. This time it did. Maybe it was because DJ and I had a "thing" going on.

Over the course of my tenure on Pediatrics, there have been six toddlers who have had to sit on my lap during music therapy group – not because they were screaming, just because they needed to. These kids reach into an even more tender area of my heart, and I remember them forever.

DJ developed a very bad type of pneumonia common to AIDS patients and ended up on a vent in the PICU. He was eventually placed on an oscillator vent, which is the jackhammer of the PICU. It is noisy and violent and it was hard to watch my friend on that piece of equipment for five weeks. During that time, everyone wondered why this child with AIDS, who was hospitalized so frequently for horrible infections, wasn't being made a DNR while in this condition. Even his aunt felt heroic measures were not appropriate. But the intensive care doctor felt that DJ could conceivably survive this disease and return to his previous state of health, which, of course, was still AIDS. Keep in mind that this was in the days before the current wonder drugs were developed – when people were routinely and horribly dying of AIDS.

Every day I went to sing to and talk to my friend in the PICU, even though he was deaf and heavily sedated. Every day I wondered why on earth we were prolonging the suffering of this child who was doomed to a terrible disease anyway. Then one day DJ was removed from the oscillator vent and placed back on the regular vent. A few days later, the PICU nurse told me they were beginning to lighten his sedation as his lungs were healing. I leaned close to DJ and put my finger in his hand. He seized my finger and opened his eyes. Those big brown eyes that I hadn't seen for five long weeks were looking back at me again. I started to cry, but couldn't even grab a tissue because DJ wouldn't let go of my finger.

DJ recovered from his pneumonia but then had to go on the inpatient rehabilitation service to build up his strength again. Eventually he progressed from maneuvering his wheelchair around the floor to running down to the playroom for the music therapy group. That's when you know it's time for kids to go home. That and when they're well enough to really start annoying staff! Then, a miracle occurred. The new anti-AIDS drugs became available and were successful for DJ. He is now living happily with his family and rarely makes an appearance at the hospital. See how wrong we all were?

Burn unit

Through the rumor mill at the hospital I heard about a two-year-old boy who had been brought in by helicopter with second and third degree burns over 98 per cent of his body. I have to admit that my first reaction was to pray that he would die. I'd been on the burn unit long enough to know what was involved in people recovering from such traumatic burns, and 98 per cent of a tiny little body is a lot. My own personal belief is that the worst day in heaven is better than the best day on the burn unit, so for the first several weeks of his hospital stay I prayed for a peaceful end to his suffering.

Then the nurses called the Child Life office to refer this little guy to me. See how effective my prayers are? So then my philosophy became – if they have made the decision that he has to live, it is our responsibility to make sure his life is worth living. I went down to the burn unit to talk with the nurses and meet this child. The fire was started when Matthew's eight-year-old brother was playing with matches in the hallway of their trailer. The parents were napping at the time. When the carpet caught fire, the older brother jumped out of a window, the five-year-old sister got scared and hid in a closet (she suffered mostly smoke inhalation), but little Matthew was developmentally delayed. At two and a half years old he still wasn't crawling. He caught the brunt of the fire before a neighbor passing by was able to pull the children out. The parents got out on the other side of the building.

Matthew's room on the burn unit was the farthest away from the nurses' station. He was wrapped completely in gauze, head to toe. His arms were in airplane traction (straight out like wings), and his legs were splayed out. He had a tracheostomy[1] and was on a ventilator. He was completely immobile, and he couldn't make a sound. I pulled a footstool near the bed to stand on so that Matthew could see me as I sang to him. All I could see were Matthew's eyes from deep within the bandages. At first I thought he might be crying. There is something horribly moving about a child crying on a ventilator. You know the sound he should be making, but it is a silent scream that gets swallowed by the machinery.

I talked to Matthew and I sang to Matthew. I saw Matthew every day he wasn't in surgery. He became a very challenging child for me. Since he couldn't move, and he couldn't speak, the only response he could give me was eye contact, but he was very good at that. From experience I knew that two-year-olds with such a high level of acuity (severity of illness/injury) typically would be able to focus with me for only short

---

1   Tracheostomy: a surgical procedure that cuts a hole into the outside of the throat. A plastic ring is inserted into the hole to keep it open and to attach to the ventilator.

periods of time. But Matthew's eyes would lock onto mine for 45 minutes easily. I was always the one who had to break it off. Matthew's sister had been discharged from the burn unit after a few weeks. Her parents came and took her home, but they never came back to visit Matthew. They eventually gave him up completely. He was a truly desperate little boy.

One day while I was singing to Matthew his eyes couldn't focus on mine. In fact, they went all over the place. By this time, I was familiar with Matthew's behavior, as limited as it was, and I knew something was very unusual and very wrong. His nurse that day was a float – someone who routinely works all over the hospital. She'd never met Matthew before. I tried to explain to her that this was very different behavior for him and that something was very wrong. I believed he was in terrible pain. She was not a usual burn unit nurse and she couldn't appreciate what I was telling her. The other nurses were busy with their critically ill patients. I went back to Pediatrics and talked with our Clinical Nurse Specialist (CNS) who is also our pain guru. She suggested I talk with the CNS for the ICUs. I did. Luckily I knew both of these women from lunch and meetings and working together on projects, so I didn't just seem like some pain-in-the-neck music therapist, although I certainly am. The Pediatric CNSs are especially attuned to children, but the patients on the burn unit were a mixed bag of children and adults. Some of the nurses were clued into children, but not all of them. The unit also functioned as an entity unto itself and was not especially open to suggestions from people outside the unit.

The Pediatric CNS for the ICUs went down to the burn unit, reviewed Matthew's chart and tactfully made suggestions for his care. The next day, Matthew was in a new room – right across from the nurses' station. He was also assigned a couple of primary nurses, who got to know him and soon fell in love with him. He was much more calm, and again his eyes locked onto mine while I sang to him. Matthew spent eight months with us and then was transferred to another children's hospital for inpatient rehabilitation. In total, he spent 18 months in hospitals. Then, by some miracle, he was adopted by a loving family who lived on a farm and had adopted two other burned kids.

Over a year later, Matthew appeared in our playroom with his new mom, coming in for contracture release surgery.[2] I knew this child had to be Matthew, but it was hard to recognize him. From being in hospitals for so long, he'd had his pressure garments[3] on consistently. (Parents at home get tired of fighting with their kids over wearing the pressure garments, and frequently become lax in enforcing them. Nurses don't have this problem – they force the kids into wearing them.) Matthew had received extremely good care, so he looked awfully good for a child with such an intense burn. His mom said he was using a walker to ambulate, but today he was a little nervous and clung to her while he watched the other kids play. I introduced myself to his mom and said that I'd worked with Matthew when he was at our hospital. She said that Matthew loved music. I took that as a compliment. After all, I would've felt completely responsible if she'd told me, "Matthew screams whenever he hears music!"

It dawned on me that perhaps my prayers weren't as ineffective as I'd thought.

---

2   Contracture release surgery: Scar tissue tends to rebuild to excess and becomes problematic when it grows between joints (elbows, fingers, knees, etc.). Contractures can pull up on affected muscles, decreasing range of motion of the joint involved, and so are surgically removed when they become too restrictive.

3   Pressure garments: These are carefully measured garments that fit tightly over the skin of burn patients in an effort to discourage excessive scar tissue rebuilding. They need to be worn 24 hours/day, removed only for eating and bathing.

10. There Are All Kinds of Suffering

Pain and fear

I hate pain. I have enormous respect for people in pain. Being blessed with migraines I sometimes walk that same path. Pain changes your life, not usually for the better. I also have enormous respect for the doctors and nurses who try to combat pain in children. Pain has historically been the most under-treated problem in hospitals. Now, at least at my hospital, it is being taken very seriously. Pain is now considered "the fifth vital sign" and is routinely checked throughout the day on each patient. Pain is currently defined as, "Whatever the patient says it is, whenever and wherever she or he says it is." We don't try to second-guess a patient's pain. Some of our kids with sickle cell anemia are in chronic pain. They somehow learn how to live with it from early childhood. Even when they're in the playroom having fun, they may still be in some amount of pain. It's a part of their life. Although we can make observations on someone's pain, it's inappropriate for us to make judgments on another's pain. They are the ones actually experiencing the sensation. It is also not uncommon for sickle cell patients to appear fine one moment, and then quickly deteriorate into severe pain the next.

Hospitals have an impressive arsenal of medicines for fighting pain. Sometimes for us, it's a matter of acting as patient advocate to make sure those medicines get to the patient (polite pain-in-the-neck music therapist). Other times the problem involves the unworkable combination of fear and pain. Fear and pain are overwhelming in any circumstance. They also overwhelm the action of many drugs, since these drugs are designed primarily to deal only with pain.

It is a common occurrence for children to be so afraid of an upcoming procedure that their pre-medications don't work. A parent once described to me giving her child Valium (an anti-anxiety med) before getting into the car and driving an hour to a clinic appointment for a bone marrow aspiration. This was in the bad old days when kids were given a local anesthetic for this procedure, which was woefully inadequate. Instead of being calm, the child fairly clung to the roof of the car like a cat as they approached the hospital. At the clinic the child had to be held down for the procedure, and then afterwards slept for the next six hours. This has become less of a problem since the oncology clinic started booking hours in one of the rooms in the Ambulatory Surgery Center. This way our kids can be given strong pain medicine while their heart and breathing rates are monitored whenever they undergo bone marrow aspirations[1] and lumbar punctures.[2] Now our patients come in knowing they'll be put out for the procedure. We have new meds that are very fast acting, very strong, with a short recovery time. These kids are in and out for these procedures, and everyone is much less anxious.

Smaller types of fear are much easier to distract children from. Often children are terrified of the nurse removing the IV. They fear it will hurt as much coming out as it did going in. Any child staring at the IV site and the nurse can easily build up fear that will increase pain. Now some children need to look. They want control, they don't want surprises, and those wishes are honored. But many children will have a better time

1   Bone marrow aspirations: A procedure used to diagnose cancers, and to determine if cancer has spread to the bone marrow. A long, large gauge needle is pushed into the pelvic bone to withdraw cells for study under the microscope.

2   Lumbar puncture: Also known as spinal tap, a procedure where a needle is inserted between the lower vertebrae of the spinal column to draw out cerebral spinal fluid. Used frequently in diagnosis for meningitis and cancers. Can also be used in administering chemotherapy (known as "intrathecal").

playing a keyboard with one hand while the nurse is working on the other. There is also the "hurry up and wait" phenomenon that can escalate fear and pain. The nurse comes into the room to draw blood, the child gets anxious, the nurse goes out of the room because she forgot something, comes back in, goes out again to get someone else's opinion about which vein to attempt, comes back in – you get the idea. This is routine, unfortunately, and can build up unnecessary fear, which, in turn, will escalate any pain. As music therapists, we can deal with fear.

I gave birth twice, using natural childbirth. No drugs – deep breathing and a husband who turned out to be a great labor coach got me through both times. I'm not talking about popping out little premature five-pounders, either. My first baby weighed in at 9 lb. 1 oz, and took nearly three and a half hours of pushing to get her out (after 15 hours of hard labor). My second baby was only 8 lb. 6 oz and I shot him nearly across the room. The point is that taking classes in prepared childbirth educated me on what to expect from the birth process, and how to trust that my body knew what it was doing. I just needed to get out of its way. (There was a delicate half-hour, however, when my body said, "*push!!*" but my doctor said, "Don't push yet." This conversation went round and round, becoming more desperate with each repetition. The uterus is the strongest muscle in a woman's body, and you don't want to run into a mad one in a dark alley. You want to stay on its good side. I describe this little half-hour from hell – known as "transition" – as the time my uterus chased me around the room while I made the sign of the cross and yelled, "Back! Back!") Natural childbirth classes helped get rid of my fear, so that all I had to deal with during birth was pain.

Now pain is brilliant at getting the body all riled up and anxious. The lungs are easily intimidated by pain and they start the process off with shallow breathing. Blood cells flowing through the lungs pick up less oxygen, and then go to the muscles. The muscles respond by tightening up, and soon a general panic alarm is set off throughout the body. Deep breathing can counteract that pain cycle immediately. If you can get a child to breath with you, face to face, and gradually slow the breathing down, the anxiety alarms will also slow down. Deep breathing is a very simple exercise that works. It is very effective for dealing with short-term pain, such as blood draws.

Guided imagery

Guided imagery, or directed imagery with music, is also very effective for pain and can provide a valuable tool for frightened children, especially teenagers. Once I received a call from the adult oncology nurse specialist. She had an 18-year-old woman with relapsed leukemia. This patient had been treated by our Pediatric service originally, but it was in the years before I'd started working at the hospital. She was heading for a bone marrow transplant as soon as they got her into remission. The problem was that Lindsey had an Omaya[3] reservoir placed in her brain through which the doctors injected chemotherapy. This wasn't painful, but she could actually hear the fluid rushing around in her brain, which made her extremely anxious and also affected her equilibrium. They'd done this procedure the day before and it had required six nurses to hold this patient down. This nurse requested that I try guided imagery with her.

I met with this young woman and her mother in the hour before the scheduled procedure. The patient was lying in bed, looking as stiff as a board. I introduced myself and described the simplified guided imagery process for them. Since I was scheduled to be somewhere else during the actual procedure, I asked the mother to watch me so she could help her daughter at the appointed time. After all, simple guided imagery and deep breathing are techniques that are available to everyone to use. I asked Lindsey to do some deep breathing with me. She agreed, but as we tried it together she barely appeared to be breathing at all. Still I encouraged her to take an even bigger breath. She was so terrified that her chest barely moved. I thought – this is not going to work at all. She seemed incapacitated by her fear.

I showed her the tape I'd brought. I have a favorite composer who works nearby in the foothills of the Sierra Nevada Mountains. David Blonski is a flautist who is extremely supportive of music therapy. He combines orchestral music with sounds of nature. His *Dance of the Dolphin* (Blonski 1986) is one of my favorites to use in guided imagery. It also turned out to be the perfect choice for a woman who is tormented by water sounds. (I hoped that the pleasant ocean sounds would drown out

3   The Omaya reservoir is surgically placed under the skull. It provides direct access for chemotherapy to be injected into the central nervous system.

the terrifying fluid sounds of the chemotherapy.) Lindsey put on the headphones and smiled at the music. I grew a little hopeful. We practiced deep breathing with the music, and I suggested she imagine herself at the ocean, perhaps on a boat, watching the dolphins and whales surfacing nearby. I told her that this ocean was perfectly safe, that she was in control, and the animals were friendly and interested in her. Lindsey closed her eyes and smiled. We worked together for an hour, and then I had to leave. The next day I got a call from the adult oncology nurse specialist. She said that the second series of chemotherapy injections for Lindsey had been a night-and-day difference from the first. Lindsey was able to hold still by herself and was completely calm. She was also extremely proud of herself. The nurse specialist said that they finished one aspect of the injections, but then realized they had to do some more. Lindsey said, "Wait a minute! Let me get my headphones!" and there was no problem. Apparently all Lindsey needed was a tool to help her cope with a difficult situation. Guided imagery and a watery tape provided that tool for her.

Cancer treatment changes

It's interesting for me to read studies involving oncology patients from the 1980s because treatment has already changed dramatically in the 16 years I've been working on Pediatrics. The nausea and vomiting induced by chemotherapy have been decreased by a wonderful new anti-emetic. Now outpatients come to the outpatient clinic for chemotherapy and stop off for a burrito on their way home.

Leukemia treatment has also changed over the last 16 years. The kids used to be hospitalized periodically over the course of a year before they went to outpatient status. Now it seems that they're diagnosed, and suddenly we're singing the last in-house chemo song six months later! This is a wonderful improvement. Families return home and to normal life much sooner these days. Hospitalization is not quite so intrusive into their lives.

Another development that will probably change again soon is the policy on isolation. This has swung back and forth in pendulum fashion since the early days of treating childhood cancers. At first, children were isolated from their families, and visiting hours were on the weekend, if you can believe it. Then kids getting chemotherapy were isolated in their rooms because the immune system is suppressed by the medicine, leaving the patient wide open to any bacteria that come along. That philosophy is very hard on the kids, and our oncologists made the call that the detrimental effects of isolation on the patients outweighed the benefits. So we reversed our isolation philosophy. Now the playroom is off limits to anyone with a runny nose, or who may be remotely infectious to our compromised kids. Visiting children are screened by the charge nurse and given a sticker on their shirts to prove they are safe for the playroom. Oncology kids with very low blood counts frequently stay in their rooms anyway, because they're feeling so lousy, and their parents are fairly nervous about exposure to other kids. But they are free to go out of the rooms when they feel up to it.

A word to parents – you know who you are

A nurse friend told me after she had children, "Being a nurse doesn't make me a better mom. Being a mom makes me a better nurse." When I came back from maternity leave, I found that I couldn't walk past a crying baby without trying to comfort her. Being a mom, I've logged several hours trying to calm my own babies after vaccinations and during high fevers (to which my daughter was prone – I want a t-shirt that says, "I survived 105°"). So I have a much bigger repertoire to draw from than before I had kids of my own.

Becoming a parent is the biggest education you'll ever get, but you also get a taste of what it would mean to lose a child. Therefore, although parenthood gives you a leg up in working with children and families, you're also more vulnerable. Every once in a while, we'll get a child who looks like one of my kids, or acts like them, or shares a name with my kids. And if they don't resemble my kids, I have 11 nieces and nephews for them to take after. I've had problems working with kids who were the same age as my kids. As a parent I can say that it's far more painful to be working on Pediatrics when you have kids of your own at home.

You're also more likely to be a little bit neurotic about illnesses. "Medical Student's Disease" occurs when new med students read about various diseases and become convinced they have them all. The same can occur among hospital staff members. We constantly see vague symptoms in kids that seem benign but then balloon into terrible diagnoses. It's easy to get just a touch whacko about our own kids. My doctor has plastered "Mom works at the Medical Center" all over my children's charts. Since most of the doctors in her practice trained at the same Medical Center, they know that I'll be calling fairly often with symptoms that scare me. Part of the problem is that cancer in adults may take 20 years to become dangerous, but cancers in children tend to explode. Children are hard-wired for growth. Since everything about them is designed to grow, cancers get dangerous very quickly in children. Often by the time they come to us, the cancer is advanced and hard to treat. I, personally, would like my kids to get a full-body MRI at their yearly physicals. I just don't think that's too much to ask. Of course the Health Maintenance Organisations tend to balk at paying $10,000 just to see if everything's okey-dokey.

There are also very scary bacterial infections that start off with "flu-like symptoms," and then become headlines for sensational newspapers like the *National Enquirer* – "Flesh-Eating Bacteria!!!" There is a tiny little window of opportunity in the beginning of these dreadful diseases when, given the right antibiotics, everyone lives happily ever after. Unfortunately, since "flu-like symptoms" are rather broad and generic, most of the medical community will make people wait until it's too late. The nurses and I just look at each other and wonder, "How can we possibly be normal parents?" We know too much. Actually we know just enough to be constantly afraid. We can make ourselves really neurotic if we're not careful.

Then there's the trauma angle. I insist that I, or my husband, drive for all our children's field trips. Now this little phobia makes me very popular with teachers and Girl Scout leaders, but it drives my husband crazy. We buy safe cars and we're fairly safe drivers, and I'm not going to let my favorite kids in the whole wide world get into an unsafe car with an unsafe driver. Unfortunately, I also cannot let my husband drive both my kids virtually anywhere without me. It's not that I don't trust him. But from working in a trauma center, I've seen many families wiped out in car accidents. One of my biggest fears is surviving the loss of my family. I'm going with them.

My husband thinks there should be a support group for spouses of Medical Center employees.

11. Complaint Department

Complaints? Moi?

I find myself in a position these days where I hear complaints about music therapy. Since we are not that common, when people meet one music therapist, they assume that person is representative of all of us. It's important that the public gets a positive impression of us.

1. A Child Life specialist from a children's hospital called me and asked why should they hire a music therapist at all. They already had a visual artist-in-residence who was urging them to hire a musician-in-residence instead of a music therapist. It sounded like the classic prejudice from college: real musicians go into performance, and the worst musicians become music therapists. Of course, these folks don't attend American Music Therapy Association conferences where music therapists routinely show off their considerable talents in the cabaret. But it helped to tell them that my intern and I had both completed bachelor degrees in performance before returning to school to pursue music therapy. We qualified as real musicians, but were also qualified music therapists.

2. This same Child Life specialist went on to describe how a music therapist had written up a proposal to work at this children's hospital as a consultant. When she told me the consultant wanted to charge $60/hour, she actually laughed

out loud. I heard a door slamming shut on a potential music therapy program in a children's hospital. The Child Life person continued, "Do you know how much money I make?" Yep, I do. I work in the Child Life department and we are among the lowest paid professionals in the hospital/city/ country/hemisphere.

Unlike this outraged Child Life specialist, however, I could see both sides of this problem. The independent contractor should be able to command a higher rate since she or he is saving the hospital a bundle of money in not paying benefits, and does not have even the teensy little bit of job security that regular staff enjoys. At the same time, it's hard to convince people who are making a small salary that a newcomer should be paid what seems like an astronomical sum to them.

3. This specialist also stressed that they needed someone who could fill in for Child Life duties as necessary, i.e., run the playroom, go to the operating room with patients, etc. They wanted someone who would not be confined to a traditional music therapy job description. Luckily I had a former intern who had gone straight from our facility to a Child Life fellowship position at Mt Sinai Medical Center in New York City. She was dual certified in music therapy and Child Life, had passed both tests, and was available. By the way, although Child Life is its own specialty, the Child Life Council allows a broad range of college majors to apply for registration. My intern found that her two degrees (in flute performance and music therapy) and a few more classes in child development were enough to qualify her. Additionally internships in Child Life require far fewer hours (480 hours) than music therapy internships so it is possible to combine the two specialties to make one more marketable. (Check out the website at www.childlife.org for more information.)

4. I also receive calls from hospitals out of my area that are looking for music therapists to provide a pilot program that they hope will grow into a real job. However they don't want

to pay private contractor prices. Their complaint is that they can only afford two hours/week of a contractor's time but want and need more hours/week to demonstrate the need for music therapy at their facility. I obviously cannot tell contracting music therapists what to do, but I respectfully suggest to new music therapists or those looking to start a pediatric program that they be willing to drop their salary down to what a hospital is ready to pay for a pilot program in the hopes of getting a foot in the door. Look at it this way – it pays better than volunteering! Perhaps you could give a "corporate discount", with the understanding that you're keeping your independent contractor rate intact, but donating your services for this specified amount of time only. Make sure you put a time limit on the pilot program – six months maximum. Specify the hours you'll be there – not too many that you'll feel ripped off, but enough to make them want more music therapy. Then prepare to knock their socks off when you show up. Be available to present inservices wherever and whenever they ask to get the word out about music therapy. Also put those hours into contact therapy time, with only the absolute minimum spent on paperwork time. In any new program there is a lot of start-up time and materials, but the nurses and patients are not going to be impressed by the amount of paperwork you do. They will be impressed and want to keep you by the hands-on music therapy you do and the difference the patients/families/staff feel when you're around.

Adagio for strings – a controlled substance

When the oncologist asks you to provide directed imagery/relaxation techniques for the highly stressed parents of a child newly diagnosed with cancer, do not use Samuel Barber's *Adagio for Strings, Opus 11* (Schirmer 1939) for background music. Although it is a truly beautiful piece, it is also the world's saddest piece of music. You might think that using the world's saddest music would "match the parents' mood," but actually it would probably increase their grief a hundredfold, which would not be the ideal response. Be very careful when working with this population. Do not make the situation worse than it already is.

Religious conversion on pediatrics

I was amazed and horrified at the first funeral I attended for a child. A hospice nurse got up and shared with the congregation how she was able to "lead Jeremy to Christ before he died." Apparently she was responsible for saving that child's soul from eternal damnation. I'm sure this was news to the child's family and pastor, as this funeral was taking place in the church the family had attended for all of the child's life. I felt this nurse was very inappropriate and unprofessional. It is crucial to respect the beliefs of the child and the family and not to force your beliefs upon your patients. I personally find the thought of manipulating a child on his deathbed to be loathsome and offensive, and told my interns at their very first interviews that I would fire them on the spot if I discovered they did such a thing.

Although I have a very deep spiritual side to my personality (it is the only thing that gets me through the process of working with dying children), it is not a belief that forces me to convince others that my way is the only way to heaven. All sorts of people come through a hospital – Sikhs, Muslims, Hindus, Old World Baptists, Mennonites, Amish, Atheists, Jews, Catholics, Buddhists, Jehovah's Witnesses, Pentecostals, etc. All these beliefs need to be respected. Sometimes, because of their dress, or dietary restrictions, I'll ask them about their beliefs. People are always happy to talk about their cultures and religions. They're grateful for my interest. I find it fascinating – remember, I'm a culture vulture. Often it will help me understand more about their family interactions and how they view health, disease, and even death. But it's *their* religion we're talking about – not mine.

Do not try to convert your patients. If it bothers you so much that children are dying who do not believe the way you do, you need to go work in another field.

Height issues, or size does matter

From working with lots of folks in wheelchairs, I am keenly aware of height issues. Towering above the person you're talking with changes the dynamics of the conversation. I have also been to lots of dog training classes in an effort to have a pet that actually graduated "Canine Good

Citizen," and I see that dominance issues are not restricted to animals that walk on four feet.

This is why I sit on the floor with scared toddlers. I had an interesting exchange with a three-year-old in the hallway once. She was wandering around, loose, no folks around, so I went up to her to see if I could help her find them. I bent down to talk with her so I'd be closer and less threatening. She saw me bending toward her, and when she answered my question, she bent over, too. Here we were in the hallway, bowing like very polite people from Japan. I saw that I would soon be lying down on the floor if we continued this conversation, so we both stood up and wandered the halls together in search of someone she knew.

If a patient is stuck in bed, you want to be in their line of sight – make sure it's comfortable for the patient, even if it isn't so comfortable for you. If they're in a wheelchair, find a place to sit also. If you think it's safe to sit on the patient's bed without causing pain to the patient, ask permission from the child first. Remember, it is invasive to sit on a patient's bed without asking first.

Dominance issues are on display among adults as well. Just watch the medical students trying to stay abreast of the attending physician as they all move in a herd through the hallways. No one wants to be in the back of the group, and they actually skip and strain to be the ones that get to walk next to their professor. This was amusing to me until I was nine months pregnant and trying to descend a flight of stairs while carrying a guitar and a bag of instruments. A mass of doctors, residents, and medical students was ascending the same flight. I hoped they would move to the side and give me room, but they couldn't give up their place next to the attending physician. I had to stop moving and cram my large barge of a body, guitar, and instruments against the wall as they pushed past me. This is not the most socially astute group of people you're likely to meet. And yes, you can imagine how indelicate a group like this can be with a terrified child. Part of our job in the Child Life department is to act as an advocate for our patients, and to help the medical staff understand and deal with these kids in developmentally appropriate ways.

Parents have their own dominance issues at play. We once had a father who was short in stature and whose son was in for a lengthy and very emotionally charged hospitalization. Doctors referred the child for psychological counseling to help him deal with anxiety and anger.

The psychologists also tried to meet with the dad for support because he was a single parent and had a history of substance abuse. The son got along well with his psych intern, but the father fled whenever he saw the psychologist coming for him. She was a big woman, much taller than him, and she always brought along a medical student who should've played professional basketball. This dad would frequently be smoking at my bus stop in the morning when I arrived. I'd sit on the bench and listen while he vented his anger and frustration from his perch, sitting on top of the backrest, his feet on the level where I sat. He told me how the "giant psychologists" would stand in front of him and behind him, and make him feel sandwiched in. This was terribly uncomfortable for him, and I was surprised the psychologists didn't pick up on this subtle but very substantial issue. It prevented this father from getting support from them.

Instead, he sought out people he felt more comfortable with whenever he needed to vent. He'd walk his son's primary nurses out to their cars after their shifts, or meet me at the bus stop. Perhaps he trusted us because we were closer to his size and he found us less intimidating.

Speaking of psychology, this dad and some patients have complained to me of the psychologists' tendency to use the phrase, "How does that make you feel?" Unfortunately, they'll ask this question of a father whose son is dying, or a teenager who is in terrible pain, and the answer always seems to be, "How the *bleep bleep blankety bleep* do you think it feels?!" Of course, they don't give this answer to the psychologists. I think they just look at the interviewer in dumbstruck horror. They tell it to me later when they're venting their anger and frustration at the intervention they've just received. So, please, use great care if you ask a question like, "How does that make you feel?" In this setting, it's pretty obvious how these events make people feel. And instead of being a support person, they'll see you as someone who just doesn't understand what they're going through.

12. Grand Finale (Finally)

Toddlers keep you humble

I love two-year-olds. They are my favorite group of people to work with. At two, kids are just becoming brave enough to venture away from mom for a while, and they're smart and curious. They love music, and I can make them laugh just by crossing my eyes. I also love babies and older kids, but toddlers are just universally mine. I work with an art therapist and a Child Life specialist who are more comfortable with teenagers – they like to talk. They like to talk like adults. I'm better with nonverbal communication so I get all the kids with cerebral palsy, all the immigrants who are new and just learning English, and all the toddlers. The thing about teenagers, however, is that since they are verbal, they let you know how grateful they are for your help. These co-workers have lots of letters from patients thanking them, letters full of love, etc. My patients can't write, can't read, some can't talk, but I do get drawings from them that I keep forever.

I had a little two-year-old girl who had a very difficult time when she was first diagnosed with leukemia. She had many complications from her chemotherapy and other medicine. She was not happy, very sick, afraid and miserable. We spent a lot of time together over the course of months. Our friendship eventually grew to the point where she went completely berserk (with joy) if I entered the playroom while she was sitting at the table. We were important to each other. Then she was finally discharged and was home for six months before she had to return to the hospital for a single day admit. Now, six months is an eternity in the life of a two-year-old, but I saw her name on the census and ran to her room to see her. We had a great time together, but on my way out of her room I heard her ask, "Mommy, who is that lady?" Working with little kids keeps you humble. I'll remember them, but they won't remember me.

Survival tips

How do you know if you're cut out for this line of work? You don't. Before I began working on Pediatrics I remember asking someone, "What is Child Life?" The answer was, "They work with dying kids." Well, I thought, I could *never* do that. I know myself well enough to know I could never stand that kind of job. Isn't that funny? Here I am, 16 years later, still thinking this is the most fun I've ever had in my life.

Of course, whenever I lose a child that I've loved for a long time I think, *I am not even remotely qualified to work here.* I used to worry that my young children would tell their day care workers, "My mommy cries all the time." I do cry. A few times I think I've even hit depression over this job. But it's never lasted more than a week or two, and eventually the joy of the work crowds out the sorrow. Music is after all, very healing and just singing together with children in the group helps me to recover. Kids are also physically demonstrative and are frequently comfortable enough to give me a hug or a kiss, a smile or a laugh, and my soul begins to heal.

Another technique that I rely on is keeping a scrapbook. I save drawings, letters from kids and families, funeral programs, everything. When I'm down and running on empty, I pull out my scrapbook and remember kids and families who were important to me. It works. Having something physical helps a lot.

I also save little pins that patients give me. My name badge is currently carrying 12 souvenirs – angels, a gold ribbon (for pediatric cancer), a green ribbon (for organ donation), an American Music Therapy Association pin, a drum, some pins from UC Davis Children's Hospital, a wooden school bus made by a patient's grandmother, and a beaded bracelet from a teenager with cystic fibrosis. On the back is taped a four-leaf clover that a patient's mother found growing outside the hospital. Next to it is a paper jack-o-lantern that a child made for me one Halloween with matching pumpkin earrings that I wore all day taped to my ears. Each souvenir that is given to me by a child or a family becomes a sort of talisman – by wearing them, part of me believes I'm helping to keep that child alive, or at least, his or her memory alive.

I write a lot for my own personal therapy. I put down on paper my grief and frustration, the anger and unfairness that I feel and witness in working with critically ill children. I also document that these children lived, that they were important, that they touched so many, and were loved by so many. It helps me cope with the unanswerable questions: Why do children have to suffer? Why do children die?

I also seek community. I work with the very best nurses on the planet. They are loving and supportive and we all constantly hold each other up. In recent years I joined a spiritual community in my town – the Religious Society of Friends (Quakers). I was drawn to their philosophy of peace in this time of war, and one benefit of their service is that I have to sit in silence for an hour each week. The first time I was there, forced to sit in silence for an hour, I thought I was going to die! But now I can easily fill the time. I do a centering exercise, send energy to those I'm worried about, and usually slip into a trance state. I always leave feeling rejuvenated. That hour forces me to sit quietly and replenish myself, something I have never made time for in my life.

Again, if you are a person who is plagued with a tendency toward depression, or have the least tiny bit of hypochondria (!), don't work on Pediatrics. It is not the environment for you! But, if you're like me, and happen to land in Pediatrics because it was the only place in the hospital who offered to give you a home, go with it for a while and see if you love it. Give it some time to discover if you can live there. Just maybe it'll become your niche – a place where you can use all of your skills, all of your humor, and all of your love. Working on Pediatrics pushes me constantly – professionally, personally, ethically. It is an environment that never ceases to educate me. It brings me sadness but also great joy. Just like home.

Coda

Pediatrics is a different realm – a place for the brave and the lucky. I'm often asked, "How can you work in such a depressing place?" Are they kidding? I work in Disneyland! Admittedly, the bad parts of my job are very bad indeed. But the good parts are so good that I can honestly say they outweigh the bad. And when a child sees me in the hallway and yells for me to come and see her, or a little one clings to my leg or climbs into my lap, or a teenager asks his nurse, "Is that head fun lady with the guitar here yet?", I know this is the best job in the entire world. Some families have told me that I should be a stand-up comic. I guess they think that working with dying children isn't stressful enough – that bombing in front of a live audience of grown-ups is just what my life needs. But I feel that if I can get a child to laugh in the hospital, I've accomplished a great deal. This has got to be one of the toughest audiences in the world. It's also the only audience I want.

One afternoon I was running off the Pediatric floor, as usual, late for my bus. As I ran past a room, I heard a five-year-old buddy of mine yell, "Bye bye, Kathy! I love you!" I stopped, walked back to the room and said, "Bye bye, Davey. I love you, too." As I raced for the bus I wondered, how many jobs are there where the people you work with yell, "Bye bye, I love you!" when you go home for the day? Not many. Pediatrics is truly special. And I am the luckiest person in the world.

References

Adam, A. (1843) "O Holy Night". Lyrics by P. Cappeau, translated and published by J.S. Dwight.

Bernstein, L. (1993) [1983] "I love you" (recorded by Barney) Capitol. (Written in 1983)

Barber, S. (1931) "Adagio for Strings, Opus 11". G. Schirmer Inc.

Blonski, D. (1986) "Dance of the Dolphin". Timeless Productions.

Cogan, R., Cogan, D., Waltz, W., and McCue, M. (1987) "Effects of laughter and relaxation on discomfort thresholds." *Journal of Behavioral Medicine 10*, 139–143.

Cousins, N. (1979) *Anatomy of an Illness as Perceived by the Patient.* New York: Bantam Books.

Cousins, N. (1983) *The Healing Heart.* New York: Avon Books.

Dillon, K. and Baker, K. (1986) "Positive emotional states and enhancement of the immune system." *International Journal of Psychiatry in Medicine 15*, 1, 13–18.

Fry, W. (1977) "The respiratory components of mirthful laughter." *Journal of Biological Psychology 19*, 39–50.

Hassed, C. (2001) "How humor helps keep you well." *Australian Family Physician 30*, 1, 25–28.

Hill, M. and Hill, P. (1935) [1934] "Happy Birthday". Clayton F. Summy Company. (Written in 1934)

Kelly, R. (1996) "I Believe I Can Fly". Jive.

Myers, J.E. and Freedman, M. (1953) "Rock Around the Clock" (recorded by Bill Haley and His Comets) Myers Music USA.

Rodgers, R. and Hammerstein, O. (1959) "My favorite Things" (recorded by the original cast of *The Sound of Music*.) Columbia CK.

Takahashi, K., Iwase, M., Yamashita, K., Tatsumoto, H., Ue, H., Kuratsune, H., *et al.* (2001) "The elevation of natural killer cell activity induced by laughter in a crossover designed study." *International Journal of Molecular Medicine 8*, 645–650.

Thompson, R. and Stanford, G. (1950) *Child Life in Hospitals: Theory and Practice.* Springfield, IL: Charles C. Thomas, Publishers.

Thorson, J. and Powell, F. (1993) "Relationships of death anxiety and sense of humor." *Psychological Reports 72*, 1364–1366.

Webber, A.L. (1993) "The Phantom of the Opera".

Wood, L. and Scott, L. (1954) "Five Little Freckled Frogs".

Further Reading

Bombeck, E. (1990) *I Want to Grow Up, I Want to Grow Hair, I Want to Go to Boise.* New York: Harper Paperbacks.

Broyles, B. (1997) *Nursing Care of Children: Principles and Practice, Clinical Companion for Ashwill and Droske.* Philadelphia: W.B. Saunders Co., The Curtis Center.

Doka, K. (1995) *Children Mourning, Mourning Children.* Bristol, PA: Hospice Foundation of America.

Foley, G. (1990) 'Care of the child dying of cancer: Part I.' *CA – A Cancer Journal for Clinicians 40,* 6, 327–354.

Gaes, J. (1987) *My Book is for Kids With Cansur – A Child's Autobiography of Hope.* South Dakota: Melius Publishing Corp.

Gaynard, L., Wolfer, J., Goldberger, J., Thompson, R., Redburn, L., and Laidley, L. (1998) *Psychosocial Care of Children in Hospitals: A Clinical Practice Manual.* Rockville, MD: Child Life Council.

Grollman, E. (1974) *Concerning Death: A Practical Guide for the Living.* Boston: Beacon Press.

LaMontagne, L. (1990) 'Stress and coping of parents of children in a Pediatric Intensive Care Unit.' *Heart Lung 19,* 4, 416–421.

Lorenzato, K. (1990) 'Grief: experiencing the death of a favorite patient.' *Music Therapy Perspectives 17,* 2, 102–103.

McConnell, L. (1983) 'Music therapy: meeting the psychosocial needs of hospitalized children.' *Journal of the Association for the Care of Children's Health 12,* 1, 29–33.

Morse, M. (1990) *Closer to the Light – Learning From the Near-Death Experiences of Children.* New York: Ivy Books, published by Ballantine Books.

Munro, S. (1978) 'Music therapy in palliative care.' *CMA Journal 119,* 9, 1029–1034.

Newman, J. (1995) *Pediatric Nursing.* Springhouse, PA: Springhouse Corporation.

Stein, S. (1974) *A Hospital Story – An Open Family Book for Parents and Children Together.* New York: Walker and Co.

Song Books

Cassidy, N. and Cassidy, J. (1986) *The Book of Kids Songs – A Holler-Along Handbook*, Palo Alto, CA: Klutz Press.

Cassidy, N. and Cassidy, J. (1986) *The Book of Kids Songs, 2*. Palo Alto, CA: Klutz Press.

The Raffi Singable Songbook: A Collection of 51 Songs from Raffi's First Three Records for Young Children (1980). New York: Crown Publishers, Inc.

The 2nd Raffi Singable Songbook: 42 Songs from Raffi's Albums Baby Beluga, Rise and Shine, and One Light, One Sun (1986). New York: Crown Publishers, Inc.

Blonski, D. (1986) *Dance of the Dolphin*. Available in audiotape and CD by A TimelessProduction, 5050 Traverse Creek Road, Garden Valley, CA 95633.

Resources

Centering Corporation is a nonprofit organization dedicated to helping people heal after bereavement. Founded by Joy and Dr Marvin Johnson in Nebraska in 1977, the organization now publishes a catalog of 150+ books and other grief resources. They also present workshops nationally that I have found very helpful: www.centering.org

The National Cancer Institute offers a wealth of information for patients and health care professionals dealing with cancer. Publications are available from their website: www.cancer.gov/cancerinfo

The Association for Applied and Therapeutic Humor provides an interesting website whose mission statement is "to advance the understanding and application of humor, laughter and play." They cover a broad spectrum of specialties including medicine, education, business and even spirituality: www.aath.org

The Laughter Remedy was created by Paul McGhee, Ph.D., an early researcher in the study of humor in medicine. After 22 years of research he now offers programs on the implementation of humor and stress management to businesses, hospitals, and other organizations. One subheading on the website is called "Humor your Tumor," and is devoted to patients dealing with cancer, their loved ones and cancer survivors: http://laughterremedy.com

The British Society for Music Therapy "aims to develop and promote music therapy. It acts as an advisory body and is a centre of information and dissemination of services, training, bibliography and research": www.bsmt.org

The Association of Professional Music Therapists provides lots of information on the field of music therapy, as well as a list of accredited universities, and people to contact for questions: www.apmt.org

Commonly Used Medical Abbreviations

$\bar{c}$
With

$\bar{s}$
without

c/o
complains of

D/C
discontinue, or discharge from hospital

dsg
dressing

△
change (as in dsg. △)

HOB
head of bed

I & O
input and output (how much a patient eats and voids). If the medical and nursing staff are keeping track of "strict I & O", you must be sure the child gets back to his bathroom in order to pee in his measuring receptacle situated in the toilet.

I.M.
intramuscular

IV
intravenous

Ⓛ
left

Ⓡ
right

Ⓑ
bilateral

N & V
nausea and vomiting

noc.
Night

NPO
(nil per os) nothing by mouth

NKDA
none known during admission (regarding allergies)

O2
oxygen

$\bar{p}$
after (post)

PERRLA
pupils equal, round, react to light and accommodate

plt
platelets

p.o.
(per os) taken by mouth

136

post-op
post-operative (after surgery)

pre-op
prior to surgery

prn
when necessary

pt.
Patient

$\bar{q}$
every

q.d.
every day

q.h.
every hour

bid
twice/day

tid
three times/day

qid
four times/day

qod
every other day

RBC
red blood cells

PRBC
packed red blood cells

PTA
prior to admission

stat
at once (emergent)

UCHD
usual childhood diseases

USH
usual state of health

UTD
up to date (regarding vaccinations)

WBC
white blood cells

Index

This index is in word by word order. The letter 'n' following a page number indicates a text note